THE BLUEPRINT
TO OPTIMIZE YOUR
IMMUNE HEALTH

11 Proven Ways to Prevent Allergies, Autoimmune and Chronic Diseases

Seni O

Contents

Disclaimer

Before you read this book, I feel that it is very important for me to fully disclose the fact that I am not a medical professional. Therefore, I caution you to consult with your doctor or a medical professional before acting upon any of the advice that I will be giving you in this book.

Having said that, I also want to make it very clear that everything written in this book has been well researched. I encourage you to check out the source materials for yourself to satisfy any concerns you may have about the advice that you are being given in this book.

Lastly, I would strongly encourage you to join my Facebook group and leave a comment about what you thought about this book. Let me know the parts of the book that helped you or a loved one that you may have shared the information you got from this book with. You can find the link to my Facebook group at the end of this book. I would also encourage you to leave a comment about what you thought of the advice I have given to you in this book in the comments section, where you purchased this book.

Introduction
What is the Immune System?

We all know that terrible feeling when we start to feel sick. Our nose gets runny, and we begin to sneeze, and our throat becomes sore. We may even come down with a fever, or experience the chills or develop some body aches. There are many symptoms that we may experience that will leave us feeling run down and unwell. These symptoms are the result of a war that is being waged in our bodies against the virus or bacteria that has infiltrated our body.

Our immune system is the frontline soldier of our body, continually fighting off sickness and disease in a never-ending attempt to keep us healthy. It is made up of many different and intricate parts that all work in their own specific ways to either protect us from infection in the first place or to eliminate it once it has been detected from our body. Understanding the basics of each of these different systems will give us a better understanding of our immune system and why keeping it healthy is of the utmost importance for our overall health.

How Does The Immune System Work?

Our immune system can be thought of as being composed of numerous different layers. Each layer plays a different role in keeping our bodies free from disease. The outer layers play a more defensive role in keeping sickness and disease out of our body. Our immune system acts as a sword and shield. The shield keeps unwanted intruders from entering our bodies. While the sword eliminates them if they do before, they have had the opportunity to do severe damage to our body.

Skin

Most people think of our skin as the material that holds our body together. While this is true, the skin also plays a very vital role in keeping pathogens out. Our skin, when fully intact, prevents harmful bacteria from entering our body. Due to the thickness and multiple layers of our skin, bacteria and viruses can't penetrate it. Our skin also secretes specific oils that contain chemicals, such as oleic acid and lysozyme, that are hazardous to certain bacteria, breaking it down or killing it on contact.

Cilia

Cilia are found primarily in our lungs and are tiny, hairlike structures that sweep in an upwards motion to push out any foreign particles and move them back up the throat and out of the body.

Chemicals and Proteins

There are numerous different chemicals and proteins that fight off intruders throughout our body and keep our bodies healthy and safe. Some of these include:

- **Mucus** - Mucus or phlegm lines the entire respiratory tract in a thin, sticky layer. This lining helps trap bacteria and other foreign objects and keeps them from entering into the body to do more damage.

- **Hydrochloric Acid** - This strong chemical is present in the stomach and helps our bodies break down food so that it can be properly digested. However, this particular acid is also powerful enough to break down and kill many viruses and bacteria that may make it into the stomach.

- **Transferrin** - Transferrin is a blood protein whose primary function is to take iron and transport it to the cells throughout the body. One of the immune benefits of this protein is that it binds tightly to the iron molecules, which means that there is no free-floating iron in the bloodstream to help feed bacteria or viruses that also require this mineral to survive and grow. Without iron, these pathogens won't be able to grow and multiply as quickly, giving the body's immune system more of an advantage when fighting them.

- **Interferons** - Just as the name suggests, interferons interfere with viruses and slow down their ability to multiply. Many different types of interferons are produced by other parts of the body, but all work in relatively similar ways to inhibit pathogens' growth and spread.

White Blood Cells

White blood cells are also known as leukocytes and vital to our body's immune system. If an invader has managed to get past the outer barriers of our body, they will next have to deal with an attack from our body's white blood cells.

White blood cells are broken down into two different categories; phagocytes and lymphocytes. They are stored in the lymphoid organs, and when a pathogen is detected, they send out a signal for the body to produce and release more white blood cells. This is when the battle begins.

Each specific type of white blood cell has its own unique way of fighting pathogens. Some surround the invading cell and essentially eat them, some rove through the body, on the lookout for more invaders, others help remove dead or dying cells and heal wounds. In contrast, others enable the body to remember and recognize specific pathogens should the body ever come into contact with them again in the future.

Acute-phase response

The acute phase response is the next step in the war that our body has waged against the invading pathogens. While our white blood cells are working on the front line of attack, our body begins to produce a protein called interleukin, which acts as a signal, sending out messages to other parts of the body, to let them know what is going on and to bring them into the war.

One specific signal reaches the brain and triggers your metabolism, causing it to increase your body's temperature to induce a fever. Pathogens grow more rapidly at a lower temperature, so the higher the body temperature, the less the infection will spread through your body.

The liver also reacts to these signals and begins to produce an increased number of specific proteins. These proteins get to work by binding to the invading bacteria and assisting in their destruction.

Also, when interleukin is released, a message is sent to the body, instructing it to increase the production of both neutrophils and eosinophils, which both help to fight off the intruding infection.

Inflammatory response

The inflammatory response is what happens towards the end of the war. Tissues have been damaged during the fight and often become red, inflamed, painful and hot. This is a direct response to the release of macrophages. These chemicals shuttle blood to the affected area to heal and remove any remaining pathogens that may still be present. This acute inflammation is central to your body's ability to quickly heal itself from infection.

Chronic inflammation occurs when your body is continuously trying to fight off intruders in your body. Lifestyle choices like drinking, smoking and eating highly processed and unhealthy foods can put your body's immune system into overdrive. Your body will begin to view all of these things like pathogens and will continue to fight. This immune response will ultimately lead to your body fighting against itself. This is what is known as an autoimmune response. [Which is a topic that we will discuss in more detail later in chapter nine.]

Chronic inflammation is one of the leading contributors to disease, causing symptoms such as fatigue, weight gain, digestive issues, high blood glucose levels, allergies, headaches, joint pain, frequent illnesses and even depression.

Acquired Immunity

Acquired immunity occurs after your body has fought off a specific pathogen or has received a vaccine. In the future, your body will be able to recognize this pathogen through memory B cells and memory T cells and can destroy and eliminate that pathogen almost immediately and with little to no immune response.

Why is the immune system so important?

Most people want to live a long and healthy life, but that just isn't possible if we fail to prioritize our immune system's health. The foods we consume, the products we use, the amount of physical activity that we get, and the supplements that we take all play a vital role in how our immune system functions and the better it works, the healthier we will feel. A properly functioning immune system will leave us feeling and looking vibrant and full of energy. Not only will we experience fewer colds and fewer bouts of the flu, but our risk of other diseases like cancer, diabetes and arthritis will be significantly lower as well.

In the following chapters, we will take an in-depth look at the different factors that directly affect our immune system. We will look at the signs and symptoms that point to an unhealthy immune system, as well as some lifestyle changes that can boost your immunity. Lastly, I want to share some delicious recipes that you can make at home to optimize your immune system's overall health.

Optimizing your immune health will help increase your lifespan by improving the overall quality of your life.

So, what are you waiting for? Turn the page to learn the first way to boost your immune health.

Sources:
www.britannica.com/science/immune-system
www.medicalnewstoday.com/articles/320101#
www.medicinenet.com/transferrin/definition.htm
www.urmc.rochester.edu/encyclopedia
www.askdrnandi.com/chronic-inflammation

Chapter One
Listen to Your Gut

We have all heard the old adage, "Listen to your gut." It is something, no doubt, that many of us have heard before. However, most of us associate this saying with our feelings. We listen to our gut when it comes to making important life decisions, but most of us don't listen to our gut when it is talking to us about our physical health.

Did you know that our stomach and digestive tract play a crucial role in our Immune health? Most of the essential vitamins and minerals that our body needs to survive are acquired from the foods we eat and absorbed through the gastrointestinal tract. If our gut isn't working the way that it should, our body won't the nutrition that it needs to function at its best. Our gut's primary purpose is to protect us from disease and help us to help us obtain and maintain a high quality of life.

Becoming in tune with our digestive health and being aware of the symptoms of a malfunctioning gut can help us better understand our overall immunity and take steps to improve our digestion and our entire wellbeing.

Tell me about my gut

Your gut is made up of your entire digestive tract. It is essentially one very long tube that starts at your mouth and continues all the way to the very end of your anus. Your gut's primary responsibility is the breakdown of food, the absorption of key vitamins, minerals and macronutrients, and the elimination of waste.

To better understand our gut and how vital our digestive tract's health is to our overall wellbeing, let's take a look at how each individual part of our gastrointestinal tract works.

Your Mouth - The mouth is the very beginning of our digestive tract. It is the upper part of our gut and plays a critical role in the digestion of our food. Our mouth which is made up of our teeth and our tongue, which all assist in the digestion of our food. When food enters the mouth, it is broken up into tiny pieces by our teeth. This process activates our salivary glands, which help to moisten the food, turning it into a watery, slushy mixture. Our saliva also contains an assortment of different enzymes, which further break down the food we have just eaten.

Your Tongue - Your tongue is a large muscle that pushes the food particles towards the back of your throat (also known as the pharynx). When these particles hit the pharynx, they activate a wave of muscular contractions, which cause your body to start swallowing, pushing the food further back and into the oesophagus.

Your Oesophagus - Did you know that your oesophagus is almost 10 inches long? This long tube connects the pharynx to the stomach and is lined with mucous membranes and muscles. Its primary function is to transport the food you have eaten to the stomach, where it can continue to be broken down and further digested. The oesophagus moves food through a process called peristalsis, which is a downward, wave-like motion that happens when the muscles that line this tube contract. When food reaches the very bottom, it comes in contact with the lower oesophagal sphincter, which is then triggered to open, releasing the food into your stomach.

Your stomach - You may have assumed that the stomach is where most digestion occurs, but this is incorrect. The stomach's primary function in the role of digestion is to take the food we have eaten and break it down even further into a liquid substance called chyme.

Your stomach releases chemicals and enzymes such as hydrochloric acid, pepsin, amylase and lipase, which work together to break down fats, carbohydrates and proteins. Some of these chemicals are so strong that they could break down other organs in our body if they were to seep out. Our stomach has a very thick layer of mucus membrane that keeps all of these corrosive chemicals inside our stomach to prevent this from happening.

Some of the foods that we eat break down faster than others. Carbohydrates act as our body's source of fuel and are digested the quickest. This is why we get a burst of energy from eating sugary foods or why an athlete may eat a high carb meal before their next game. Proteins aid in muscle repair and production and are broken down at a medium pace while fats take a little longer.

To further help the digestion process, your stomach muscles begin to contract, swirling the food around, breaking it down even faster. When the stomach's job is finished, food slowly begins to pass into the duodenum, the first part of the small intestine.

Your Small Intestine - Your small intestine is approximately twenty feet long and is made up of three different parts: the duodenum, the jejunum and the ileum. The duodenum is connected to the stomach and is the first place that chyme arrives after leaving the stomach. Here, bile and enzymes from the liver, the gallbladder and the pancreas continue to break down the food particles. Once these particles are as small as possible, they flow from the duodenum into the jejunum and the ileum.

The function of these next two sections of the small intestine is to absorb the nutrients from the food you have eaten and shuttle them into the bloodstream, where they can be utilized by your body. The jejunum and the ileum have numerous twists, turns and folds, which increase the surface area inside, making your body able to absorb more of the nutrients it consumes. There are very fine, tiny hairs called villi and microvilli that line these parts of the small intestine, which help to trap and absorb these nutrients, pulling them into the bloodstream and facilitating their delivery throughout your body.

Once all of the nutrients have been removed, the leftover particles are moved to the large intestine, where the final stages of digestion occur.

Your Large Intestine - Your large intestine comprises four different parts: the cecum, the colon, the rectum and the anus. It is almost six feet in length. Its primary function is to absorb water, salts and electrolytes from the leftover, indigestible food particles and remove these unusable particles from the body as waste.

Your large intestine also contains an estimated 700 different bacteria species, which breaks down fiber and polysaccharides, assisting in their absorption. Also, it creates a range of different vitamins that your body needs for survival, such as vitamin B, vitamin K and biotin.

Another vital role that your large intestine plays is its production of antibodies. These antibodies are created in the lymphoid tissues, which line the large intestine and help fight harmful bacteria and improve our immunity.

As food moves through the large intestine, it becomes denser because it is absorbing water. This process can take between three to ten hours, after which time the solid faecal matter is formed in the colon. The muscles of the colon contract, pushing the faeces through the colon and into the rectum. When here, the rectum's walls expand, sending a signal to the brain which gives you the urge to go to the bathroom. When you go to the bathroom, it releases the sphincter of the anus to eliminate the leftover waste from your body.

The entire digestive process is controlled by your brain, nervous system and other hormones in the body. Together they trigger the release of gastric juices before you even start eating and send signals to different receptors in the body to facilitate the release of certain enzymes at specific times and causing contractions to further break down and digest your food.

What is My Microbiome

You may already be well aware that our entire bodies, both inside and out, are covered with the bacteria, viruses, fungi and protozoa that make up our individual microbiomes, but did you know that in total, there are over 100 trillion of them! If you were to collect all of these microbes and weigh them together, the total weight would be over five pounds.

Our microbiome can be compared to a bustling city at rush hour with organisms moving about, both inside of us and on our skin. It is a critical component of our health and wellbeing. It helps us digest the food that we eat, it protects our bodies against other bacteria and viruses that cause illness and disease, it helps to balance our hormones. It helps produce specific vitamins vital to our survival, such as B12, thiamine, riboflavin, and vitamin K.

Our microbiome is made up of both good and bad bacteria that, when in balance, live together in harmony. If our microbiome becomes out of balance, we will experience something called dysbiosis, which will make us much more susceptible to illness and disease, having a huge and detrimental effect on our immune system and can lead to a whole range of different symptoms.

Using antibiotics, eating an unhealthy diet, smoking, drinking alcohol, certain environmental factors, and lack of exercise can directly affect our microbiome. Since a vast majority of the body's immune cells reside in the gut, dysbiosis can directly impact our immune system, leading to poor health, frequent illness, and a whole host of other symptoms.

Warning Signs of an Unhealthy Gut

When your gut is not functioning at its optimal level, and your microbiome isn't flourishing as it should be, a whole host of different symptoms can present themselves. Some are obvious and can be easily associated with your digestion, but others are more elusive.

Let's take a look at some of the most commonly occurring symptoms that are directly related to dysbiosis.

- **Nausea** - This warning sign is a pretty obvious one. When we feel sick to our stomach, it's usually a pretty clear sign that something is wrong. Acute nausea and vomiting are usually a clear indication of infection. It is our body's way of trying to quickly remove bacteria or viruses that have been consumed through the digestive tract.

- Chronic nausea that persists for an extended period of time could indicate an imbalance in your microbiome, meaning that food isn't broken down, digested and absorbed as it should be.

- **Gas and Bloating** - Gas and bloating are caused by food that ferments in the digestive tract. While some level of fermentation is normal and even necessary for good gut health, too much can cause an excess of gas. This occurs when food particles are not broken down properly or are not moved through the digestive tract expeditiously. Instead of being either absorbed or eliminated, they sit and ferment, producing hydrogen, carbon dioxide and methane.

- **Bad Breath** - Halitosis, also known as bad breath, is often a clear indication that something is out of balance in your microbiome. If either the flora in your mouth or in your gut is not present in the quantities that it should be, bad breath will likely occur.

- **Weight Gain** - Certain studies have shown that people who are overweight have a higher number of enzymes present in their body's microbiome. These enzymes allow them to metabolize food at a quicker rate and specialize in hoarding away calories. These people also showed a less diverse microbiome with fewer good bacteria present in the gut.

- **Constipation** - Constipation, especially that of a chronic nature, is often the cause of an increased bacterial overgrowth in either the small or large intestine. This bacteria can cause an increase in gas production which often significantly slows down the amount of time that is required for the body to eliminate waste.

- **Diarrhoea** - When our gut microbiome is out of balance, It can result in soft stool production, which can lead to you getting diarrhoea. Suppose there are harmful bacteria or parasites present in the digestive tract. In that case, your body will do what it can to expel them as quickly as possible, which often results in you getting diarrhoea. When our bodies cannot digest food properly due to reduced microbiome health, the body has no choice but to get rid of it as waste. Diseases of the bowels, such as Crohn's or Colitis, are often closely associated with dysbiosis.

- **Heartburn** - When the microbiome in your gut is out of balance, symptoms such as heartburn can occur. Some doctors also theorize that Gastroesophageal Reflux disease (also known as GERD) is caused by an excess of certain bacteria in the small intestine. This causes the pressure from the gas build-up to force the stomach acid contents upwards, causing the disease's unwanted and uncomfortable symptoms.

- **Insomnia** - The microbes in our gut are responsible for hormone regulation and specific Inflammatory triggers that regulate our organs' functioning. When these microorganisms are not in symbiosis with each other, our organs may not function optimally, causing sleep disruptions, and there may be disruptions to the hormones that contribute to our sleep, such as serotonin and melatonin.

- **Food Allergies and Intolerances** - While the research is still ongoing, studies have shown a direct link between food allergies and the microbiome in your gut. People with specific food allergies or intolerances also tend to have imbalances in the number of good bacteria in their intestinal tract.

- **Frequent Yeast Infections** - Certain levels of yeast are normal and can be found in everyone's body. Still, when yeast bacteria continues to grow to high levels, this is called Candidiasis and is an obvious sign that your microbiome is out of balance.

- **Fatigue** - If we aren't digesting our food correctly, how can we possibly have the energy to get through our day? Having an unhealthy microbiome in our gut can lead to sleep disorders. It also means that all of the micro and macronutrients that our body needs to function aren't being adequately absorbed. This will leave you feeling tired and unable to focus.

- **Acne and Skin Problems** - Issues with our skin, such as acne, eczema and rosacea, are often caused by imbalances in our gut. Although studies are still being conducted to prove the exact relationship between our gut and our skin, it has become clear that a healthy and thriving microbiome almost always leads to healthy and radiant skin.

- **Mood Changes** - Microbes in your gut are closely linked to the activity that occurs in your brain. Whether through blood vessels, the vagus nerve or endocrine cells, your gut's microbiome can travel to the brain, having a direct effect on your mood and mental state. Studies have also found that many people who suffer from other gut-related diseases also suffer from anxiety or depression or even dementia and Alzheimers later in life.

- **Food Cravings** - Most of the food cravings that we experience are not actually coming from our minds, as most of us most likely believe. They are actually coming from our gut! The bacteria in our intestinal tract will send messages to the brain, telling it what it "needs" in order to feed your body. If your microbiome is unbalanced, then your food cravings will be unbalanced as well. If there are too many bacteria that require sugar molecules to thrive (yeast, for example), then you will find yourself craving sugar!

Do any of these signs and symptoms sound familiar? I'm sure at some point in your life, you have experienced at least one of these. Short-term, acute symptoms may not be an indicator of an overall unhealthy gut or an off-balance microbiome. Short-term symptoms may just be a direct result of something we have just eaten, that for one reason or another (perhaps spoiled food or a food sensitivity) just doesn't agree with us. It's the long-term, chronic symptoms that we need to be most concerned about. The constant bloating, heartburn, fatigue, skin issues and mood changes (to name just a few) are all warning signs that should be taken very seriously.

If not identified and treated, dysbiosis in the body can seriously compromise our health. Some of the most common diseases that are linked to an unhealthy gut include:

- Type 1 Diabetes
- Heart Disease
- GERD
- Crohn's and Colitis
- IBS
- Leaky Gut Syndrome
- Depression
- Possibly many more, the studies are still ongoing!

How is Microbiome Dysbiosis Diagnosed?

Identifying the problem is the first step in this battle. Once we have learned to listen to our gut and have become aware of everything that it is trying to tell us, we can begin to take the necessary steps to bring balance to our microbiome. If you learn to listening to and taking better care of your gut, you can significantly lower your risk of contracting a life-threatening disease.

There are many different ways that dysbiosis can be diagnosed:

- **Symptoms Check** - Your healthcare provider may look at your symptoms, the medications (especially antibiotics) that you have taken in the past and are currently taking, your eating habits, and your bowel movement habits and make a diagnosis based on their findings.

- **Stool Analysis** - A Comprehensive Stool Analysis (CDSA) can be performed to check the balance of both good and bad bacteria present in your stool and give a good indication if your gut's microbiome requires some help.

- **Hydrogen Breath Test** - This particular test measures the number of certain gasses present in your breath to determine if there is an overgrowth of specific bacteria. Your doctor will give you a sugar solution to drink and then have you blow into a type of balloon, after which your breath will be analyzed.

- **Biopsy** - This is the most invasive method to check for dysbiosis in your gut and involves your doctor taking a biopsy of a small sample of the tissue from your digestive tract and testing it in a laboratory to determine the levels of bacteria that are growing there.

If all of this sounds overwhelming, don't worry! All the information you need to know about the right foods to incorporate into your diet and the proper nutritional supplements that can increase your gut health and boost your immunity is up next!

Sources

- www.thedigester.com/how-does-the-digestive-system-work/
- www.britannica.com/science/human-digestive-system
- www.medical-reference.net/2012/07/how-does-digestive-system-work.html
- www.sciencedirect.com/topics/medicine-and-dentistry/peristalsis
- www.livescience.com/52048-small-intestine.html
- www.depts.washington.edu/ceeh/downloads/FF_microbiome.pdf
- www.hsph.harvard.edu/nutritionsource/microbiome
- https://www.ncbi.nlm.nih.gov/pmc/articles/PMC6834330/

Chapter Two
Garbage in, Garbage out

Imagine for a moment that your lifelong dream was to own a fancy sports car. It's shiny and fast and purrs like a kitten! You've invested a lot of time and money into too. Not only do you spend your spare time on the weekends polishing and cleaning it, but you also spend countless hours driving it each week. You depend on it to take you to work and the grocery store and run all of the other errands you have to run. In short, it's your pride and joy. So you want to make sure you take good care of it. You take it for regular maintenance, use premium gas when you fill it up, and only use the highest quality motor oil. You do all that you can to protect your investment to keep it looking and running at its absolute best!

Unfortunately, many of us fail to give the same level of care and attention to our bodies. Our body is an amazing machine. For our body to function at its best, we need to make sure that everything we put into it is of the highest quality. Remember the saying, "You are what you eat." If we eat a bad diet, we will have poor health, and vice-versa. Food is the fuel that keeps us fit and healthy. If we don't eat nutritious food, how can we possibly expect to enjoy optimal health?

In this chapter, we are going to look at why good nutrition is such an essential part of our overall health and wellbeing. We are also going to learn why good eating habits can change our lives.

All About Micronutrients and Macronutrients

All of the food we eat can be broken down into two main categories: micro and macronutrients. These are the building blocks for our life and our health, and without the proper balance of both of these types of nutrition, our health will suffer, and we can experience a whole range of different symptoms and, in extreme cases, even disease.

What are Macronutrients?

Macronutrients are substances that the body requires in large amounts to survive, develop and grow. They can be broken down into three categories:

- **Carbohydrates:** Over the years, due to fad diets and media hype, carbs have gotten a bad reputation, but the truth of the matter is, out of any nutrient that our body requires, carbohydrates are by far the most important. Healthy, complex carbohydrates can be found in abundance in fruits, vegetables, nuts and seeds, beans and legumes, dairy products, and starchy foods such as potatoes. Carbohydrates are easily and quickly broken down and metabolized by the body, and therefore, they are our primary energy source. They give us the fuel that we need to power through our days, and while other macronutrients also provide us with energy, carbohydrates are by far the best and fastest way to get the energy that our bodies require.

  Healthy sources of carbohydrates are also full of fiber which acts as nature's broom, helping with digestion and sweeping out all of the waste that our body produces. Carbs fuel all of our organs and keep them working as they should, and they also give our brains the power that it needs to keep us focused and thinking clearly.

- **Proteins:** Proteins are the building blocks of our cells. They are found in large amounts in meat, beans (legumes) and can be found in smaller amounts in dairy products and some vegetables. Our bodies synthesize protein to facilitate muscle repair and growth.

- **Fats:** Healthy fats that are naturally found in foods like nuts, meats, and dairy products are essential for our survival. They are a dense energy source that makes up our cell membranes and over 60% of our brain. Our body stores fats to use as an energy source in situations when carbohydrate intake is low. It is also necessary for the metabolism of all fat-soluble vitamins, like vitamin A, D, E, and K.

  Unhealthy sources of fats, also known as trans fats, do not occur naturally and are only found in highly processed foods. They are created by adding hydrogen to naturally occurring fats which hydrogenates them and gives them a longer shelf life. All too often, your body is not able to metabolize these fats properly. Therefore they act as a poison in your system, raising your bad LDL cholesterol levels and resulting in a whole host of diseases.

What are Micronutrients

Micronutrients are made up of the vitamins and minerals that our bodies require in order to stay healthy, fight disease and grow. As the name suggests, micronutrients are needed in small amounts, but it is imperative that we consume this amount of micronutrients daily. Micronutrient deficiencies can lead to a wide range of different symptoms, weakening our immune systems and eventually contracting a disease.

Some micronutrients are water-soluble, which means that they dissolve in your body's fluids and are not easily stored. Your body will flush out any excess of these vitamins through your urine. Some of the most common water-soluble vitamins include vitamin C and all of the different B vitamins.

Fat-soluble vitamins are stored in your body's fatty tissues, and it is often recommended that you take them with a healthy fat source to enhance their absorption since they require fat to be broken down in the body. As mentioned earlier, vitamins A, D, E, and K are all fat-soluble vitamins.

Minerals play a whole host of different functions in our bodies, from helping to develop our bones and teeth to balancing our fluid levels. Some are required in larger amounts, while others are only needed in trace amounts for proper functioning. Here are some examples of some minerals that our body needs to functions at its best: calcium, magnesium, iron, sulfur, zinc, potassium, sodium, and selenium.

We need to make sure that our bodies are getting a wide variety of different macro and micronutrients. Ensuring that you don't have a deficiency in any of these essential minerals is one of the first steps you need to take to gain control of your health. Feeding your body nutrient-rich food will help ensure that you have the energy required to get through the day and the nutrients needed to keep you fit and healthy.

Ditch the Fast Food

The fast-food industry began in the late 1940s and has boomed in popularity since. The food that they offer is cheap, fast, and can taste delicious. But it's no secret that fast food is bad for you. The question is why?

There are so many different reasons that fast food is bad for us. This is because it is hard to know where to even begin. Let's take a look at some of the top reasons that eating at fast-food restaurants is unhealthy:

- **Sodium** - The salt content in fast-food is extremely high. Depending on what you choose to eat, some meals may contain close to half of the daily recommended allowance in just one serving. Consuming too much sodium can have a vast number of detrimental effects on your body and can be extremely harmful to your kidneys.

- **Sugar** - Fast food is loaded with sugar! This sugar overload is terrible for your gut health, and regular consumption of high sugary foods can lead to Type 2 diabetes.

- **Calories** - Did you know that one meal from a fast-food restaurant can contain an entire day's worth of calories? This caloric overload, all at one time, can wreak havoc not only on your digestive tract but on your entire body.

- **Trans Fats** - We have already talked about the fact that trans fats are bad for us, and fast food is well known for its high levels of trans fats. Regularly eating trans fats can lead to high cholesterol, heart disease, and clogged arteries.

- **Quality of Ingredients** - To make fast food inexpensive, the ingredients used have to be affordable. To achieve this, most fast-food manufacturers use low-quality meat and produce to keep their production costs as low as possible.

- **Lack of Fiber** - Most fast-food items are very high in refined carbohydrates, which means that they are very low in fiber. This lack of fiber can cause constipation and digestive issues.

- **Lack of vitamins and minerals** - Because fast food is highly processed, it holds very little nutritional value. There are very few vitamins and minerals in most fast-food choices meaning that regular consumption will leave your body lacking in the essential nutrients that it needs to survive.

- **Addictive Properties** - Many options on a fast-food menu contain a chemical called monosodium glutamate. It is a food additive used to increase flavor and directly affects the pleasure center in the brain. When consumed, it gives you that "feel good" feeling and causes you to crave more of it.

Why Choose Organic?

We have all heard the term organic; in fact, most supermarkets that we walk into have an entire section devoted to organic foods! But what does the term organic mean, and why are organic foods the better choice?

What does the term "organic" mean?

According to the Merriam Webster Dictionary, the term organic means: "of, relating to, yielding, or involving the use of food produced with the use of feed or fertilizer of plant or animal origin without employment of chemically formulated fertilizers, growth stimulants, antibiotics, or pesticides."

When you see a product in the grocery store labeled organic, the United States Department of Agriculture (or USDA) has ensured that the product has met its specific organic certification requirements. These requirements look into certain factors such as:

- The type and quality of soil being used to grow food
- The practices used in raising and caring for animals
- Pesticide use
- The use of additives in food

Often the labeling you may see on products can get confusing. Here is a breakdown of what the different types of organic labeling mean so that you can make educated purchases in the future:

100 % Organic - This means that 100% of all of the ingredients used in the product (excluding salt and water) have come from organic sources.

Organic - When a product is labeled as "Organic," a minimum of 95% of the ingredients contained within must be from wholly organic sources. This means that up to 5% of the components can be from non-organic sources. These items can only be used if they are not commercially available in organic forms.

Made with Organic - A product labeled with specific organic ingredients must contain at least 70% organic components and will not be labeled as USDA certified.

What is GMO?

GMO stands for Genetically Modified Organism. It refers to foods that have been genetically altered in a science lab. This alteration is usually done to create greater crop yields and larger individual pieces of produce. The impact of GMO products on your health is still something that many doctors and nutritionists are split over. There have been scientific and medical studies that have been conducted and peer-reviewed articles that have been written in favor of or against GMO Foods. Due to the changes made to the product's specific genes, issues with digestion and food allergies are often present. There has been associated with increased levels of diseases and cancers.

Why is choosing organic foods important for my health?

Eating a diet that mainly comprises of organic foods is an excellent way to make sure that your body is getting a high level of nutrients from the foods that you eat and as few additives and pesticides as possible. Any chemicals included in your food will have a detrimental effect on your body and its processes.

As a side note, choosing organic foods over non-organic food has a positive impact on the environment. It helps keep the soil and our water systems free from contaminants, and it also ensures the safe and humane treatment of our farm animals.

Do I have to buy only organic foods?

If you have ever purchased organic foods before, it will come as no surprise that they are more expensive than buying regular foods. This is because the quality standards are higher for organic foods and the production measures and methods are more time-consuming and more costly as well. Unfortunately, those costs usually get passed on to the consumers, which makes choosing organic a more expensive option.

If you're working within a specific grocery budget (who isn't!), here are some tips for splurging and purchasing organic foods and when you can save a little and buy the regular variety. According to the Environmental Working Group, these foods are known as the "Clean 15," and through product testing have consistently shown that they contain the least amount of pesticides.

The Clean 15

1. Avocados
2. Sweet Corn
3. Pineapple
4. Onions
5. Papaya
6. Frozen Sweet Peas
7. Eggplant
8. Asparagus
9. Cauliflower
10. Cantaloupe
11. Broccoli
12. Mushrooms
13. Cabbage
14. Honeydew Melon
15. Kiwi

If you are looking to save a little bit of money, purchasing the regular variety of the foods that made it onto this list will help you do so.

Due to the nature of these fruits and vegetables and the farming practices required to produce them, nutritionists advise that you should be the organic variety.

Always Buy Organic:

1. Spinach
2. Dairy Products
3. Meats
4. Tomatoes
5. Strawberries
6. Pears
7. Apples
8. Peaches
9. Potatoes
10. Grapes
11. Cucumbers
12. Baby Food

Why are Superfoods Super Heroes?

You have probably heard the term "Superfood" when turning on the TV, flipping through a magazine, or taking a walk up and down the aisles of your local grocery store. This term has grown in popularity in recent years as more information is being revealed about the amazing healing properties and health benefits that some foods have. Superfoods are incredibly dense in nutrients, containing ample vitamins, minerals, and other substances that are believed to be essential for disease prevention and optimal vitality.

Here is a list of some of the top superfoods that you should start including in your diet today!

- **Berries** - Strawberries, blueberries, and raspberries are all excellent sources of nutrition. They are considered one of the top superfoods due to their high levels of vitamins, fiber, antioxidants, and phytochemicals (also known as flavonoids). These berries protect the body against free-radical damage, protect the heart and cardiovascular system, stop the development and spread of cancer, and possibly even help fight certain viruses.

- **Garlic** - Not only is garlic a great way to spice up your food. Garlic also has some considerable health benefits as well. Garlic is well known to help boost the immune system and fight off colds. It also helps lower your blood pressure, protect against heart attacks and strokes, and lower bad cholesterol in the body and protect against dementia and Alzheimer's disease. Garlic also has many antioxidants for overall health, and some studies have shown that the level of sulfur in garlic may help pull heavy metals out of the body.

- **Ginger** - Among the many different health benefits that ginger has to offer is its incredible ability to aid in digestive health. Ginger is proven to help with nausea, the digestion of food, the reduction of gas, the flow of food through the small and large intestines, and constipation. Ginger also has excellent anti-inflammatory properties removing free-radicals from the body and reducing swelling, especially around joints.

- **Turmeric** - This bright yellow seasoning is considered a superfood because it has so many properties that aid our body's overall health and wellness. Turmeric is excellent for digestion and has been thought to stimulate the gallbladder to help secrete bile to improve the digestion process. It is also a potent anti-inflammatory that can help reduce the symptoms of inflammatory conditions such as eczema, psoriasis, osteoarthritis, and irritable bowel syndrome.

- **Cranberries** - If you are looking for an excellent way to boost your overall health, adding some fresh, organic cranberries into your diet is an excellent idea! Cranberries have so many different health benefits it's hard to name just a few! They are full of vitamin C, which can help to fight viruses. They are packed full of antioxidants that can help remove free-radicals and reverse the oxidation process, reducing the effects of aging. They are also known to improve the good bacteria in your gut, helping your microbiome flourish. They can also aid in the health of the urinary tract, reducing the incidence of infection.

- **Macca** - Macca is a superfood that is derived from the root of the Siberian Ginseng plant. It is a highly effective adaptogen that boosts the immune system, balances hormones, supports the adrenal glands, and boosts overall energy levels. It is most commonly found in a powdered form and is excellent to add in shakes, smoothie bowls, or your morning oatmeal.

- **Salmon** - Most people think of superfoods as being derived from fruits and vegetables, but salmon is an excellent superfood as well. It contains a very high level of omega-3 fatty acids, which are great for both cardiovascular health and brain function. Salmon also helps with the production of melatonin and therefore helps to improve sleep. It is also loaded with B-vitamins, minerals, protein, and antioxidants.

- **Kale** - Previously almost unheard of, kale is everywhere these days, and for good reason! Kale is bursting with all kinds of vitamins, minerals, and antioxidants, making it a superfood powerhouse. It is rich in fiber, contains a whole list of immune-boosting vitamins, can help lower cholesterol, fights Type 2 Diabetes, is high in iron, and is loaded with free-radical fighting properties.

- **Acai** - Much like other types of berries, acai berries are full of antioxidants and vitamins, making them a great addition to anyone's diet, especially if you are looking to boost your immune health. They are thought to be good detoxifiers and can help reverse the effects of free-radicals in the system.

The Importance of Staying Hydrated

We have heard it many times before; drink at least eight cups or 2 liters of water every day. We know that staying hydrated is essential for good health. But why?

Our bodies are made up of approximately 60% water, and water is vital for so many of our bodily functions:

- It helps to lubricate our joints.

- It regulates our body temperature.

- It contains minerals that are essential for balancing our electrolytes.

- It makes up over three-quarters of both our lungs and our heart and ensures that they keep functioning properly.

- It helps with digestion by aiding in the absorption of nutrients.

- It detoxifies the body by flushing out waste and toxins.

What happens when we become dehydrated?

When dehydration occurs, our bodies are not able to function as they should. Acute dehydration can occur due to strenuous exercise or exposure to extreme heat for an extended amount of time. Chronic dehydration occurs when we regularly go throughout our days without consuming enough water.

Symptoms of dehydration include:

- Infrequent urination

- Dark yellow urine
- Headaches
- Dry skin
- Fatigue
- Constipation
- Digestive issues
- Skin problems
- High blood Pressure
- High cholesterol
- Electrolyte imbalances
- Joint pain
- Bladder and kidney problems
- Early signs of aging

Is all water created equal?

The short answer to this question is no. First off, let's take a look at what we mean by staying hydrated by drinking water. Many people assume that drinking any fluid will help keep them hydrated, but this isn't the case. Coffee, tea, and caffeinated beverages all act as a diuretic, pulling fluids from the body and thus causing it to become dehydrated. None of these beverages should count towards your daily water intake. If you do drink these beverages and alcohol, please do so in moderation.

Unfiltered tap water can be extremely hazardous to your health and should be avoided as well. Testing on some tap water has shown a wide variety of different dangerous chemicals, including small amounts of hormones, prescription drugs, fluoride, chlorine, viruses, and bacteria, to name just a few.

Alkaline, reverse osmosis, or purified water are the best choices of water to drink. All of these options have gone through a rigorous filtration process that removes most (if not all) of the harmful particles that can be found in regular tap water.

Now that we have a better understanding of what to eat and drink to boost our immune system, we can now move onto the next tip, which is for us to enhance our diet by taking vitamin and mineral supplements. To this end, we will be looking into some of the best immune-boosting supplements available on the market today and how taking these can improve our wellbeing and help us be better prepared to fight off illness and disease.

Sources

- www.study.com/academy/lesson/what-are-macronutrients-definition-funcions-examples.html
- www.cdc.gov/nutrition/micronutrient-malnutrition/micronutrients/index.html
- www.healthline.com/nutrition/micronutrients
- www.medhealthdaily.com/reasons-why-fast-food-is-bad-for-you
- www.ewg.org/foodnews/clean-fifteen.php
- www.merriam-webser.com/dictionary/organic
- www.ams.usda/gov/grades-standards/organic-labelling-standards
- www.nauralsociety.com/the-dangers-of-tap-water-and-how-to-protect-yourself/
- www.myfooddata.com

Chapter Three
Immune Boosting Supplements

While it would be wonderful if we could get all of the vitamins, minerals needed for optimal health from our regular diet, the sad truth is that very few people are able to get the full recommended dose of essential vitamins and minerals from food alone. Time restraints, budget restraints, and just the sheer complex task of tracking every little thing that we eat make it impossible to guarantee that we will always get the exact amount of nutrients that we need.

While eating a well-balanced diet that consists of a large portion of fruits, vitamins, and whole foods is an excellent way to add as much nutrition as possible, it is still not enough. However, adding vitamin and mineral supplements to your diet will give your immune system an extra boost. They will also ensure that any nutrients that are not contained in the food you have eaten will be included in your diet.

Which supplements should you be taking?

Vitamin C

Vitamin C plays a critical role in your immune health. It helps protect cell walls from viral attacks, scavenges the body for oxidants, and removes them. Vitamin C has microbial killing properties as well and can help rid the body of certain bacteria. Overall, a diet high in vitamin C is a great way to stay protected from illness and disease. As an added bonus, vitamin C is also great for your skin health and can help minimize the effects of aging.

Vitamin C can be found in high amounts in guavas, kiwi, oranges, bell peppers, strawberries, broccoli, tomatoes, snow peas, and kale. Rosehip tea is also an excellent source of this vitamin.

The daily recommended amount of vitamin C is 90mg.

Vitamin D3

Most people think of vitamin D as being an essential vitamin for bone health, and it is. But vitamin D offers so much more. It is imperative for proper immune function, and deficiencies in this vitamin can lead to severe illness and autoimmune diseases. Vitamin D is necessary for the effective repair of damaged cells. In fact, almost all of the cells that comprise our immune system contain vitamin D receptors, which means that vitamin D plays a foundational role in our entire immune system's development and optimal functioning.

If its immune-boosting properties aren't enough to convince you to take a daily dose of vitamin D, know that it improves your mood and combat depression. If you are an African American male, there is a solid, possibly life-saving reason you should take a daily dose of vitamin D; it lowers your prostate cancer risk. This is because African American men are unable to produce vitamin D in their bodies, unlike Caucasian men who can. The only other way that African American males can make sufficient amounts of vitamin D in their bodies is to exposed themselves to direct sunlight for at least 30 minutes a day.

The best way to get your daily dose of vitamin D is through exposure to the sun. There is a specific type of chemical on your skin converted to vitamin D when exposed to sunlight. Vitamin D can also be derived from fish and seafood, mushrooms, egg yolks, and fortified foods like milk and dairy products.

The actual amount of vitamin D that the average person requires is under debate. Some health practitioners recommend the average adult take 600IU daily, while others feel that 4000IU is needed. To find out the right amount for you, be sure to ask your pharmacist or healthcare provider.

Zinc

Zinc is a mineral that is extremely important for immune health. Studies have shown that it plays a vital role in the creation, development, and growth of immune cells, and people who are deficient in zinc often suffer from more frequent and severe illnesses. Zinc also helps reduce inflammation caused by a disease which allows your body to heal and recover faster.

Zinc can be found in beef, shrimp, oysters, spinach, kidney beans, flaxseed, pumpkin seeds, and garlic.

The daily recommended dose of zinc is 10mg.

Magnesium

Did you know that it is estimated that approximately 68% of Americans are deficient in magnesium? This mineral plays an essential role in a myriad of bodily functions, and without proper levels, it is difficult for your body to function at its best. Magnesium helps to increase the immune cell population and works on the body to decrease stress. It promotes proper adrenal function and promotes better sleep, which helps to reduce anxiety. When you are experiencing high levels of stress, your immune response is often compromised. Magnesium has also been shown to increase the absorption of vitamin C. As an extra perk for taking this mineral, you will likely experience fewer muscle cramps. Magnesium has also been known to reduce the symptoms of restless leg syndrome.

Magnesium can be found in dark chocolate, avocados, nuts, legumes, tofu, seeds, bananas, and some leafy greens.

The daily recommended dose of magnesium is 300mg per day.

Omega 3

Omega 3 is another essential supplement for overall good health. This fatty acid helps improve our cardiovascular and brain health and plays a vital role in our immune systems' health. Omega 3's are made up of three different components: ALA, EPA, and DHA. While studies are still ongoing, scientists have concluded that Omega 3's play a vital role in cell wall structures' make-up. The right balance of Omega 3's and Omega 6's in the body is essential if our immune system hopes to win its fight against a harmful bacteria or virus.

Some excellent sources of Omega 3 fatty acids are fish and seafood, nuts and seeds, and plant-based oils.

Most studies about the daily intake of Omega 3's suggest that taking a dose of 500mg should be sufficient for overall health.

Echinacea

Echinacea has been used for centuries to help fight the common cold. It contains a high level of antioxidants and can help to boost up other antioxidants that are already in the body. Studies of this plant have shown that it can help fight off viruses and the common cold, reducing its severity and duration by up to a day and a half. As an added bonus, Echinacea is also effective at lowering blood sugar levels. It also helps with mood and anxiety, reduces headaches, and is a potent antioxidant.

Echinacea is a plant that belongs in the daisy family. You can find this a supplement in the form of a pill, a tea, or a tincture.

For helping to boost your immunity and fight off an impending cold, the usual recommended dose of Echinacea is 300mg, three times a day.

Probiotics

Adding probiotics to your diet, whether through a dietary source or in pill form, is an excellent way to balance your gut microbiome and boost your overall immunity. As we have already learned in the first chapter of this book, our gut's health is critical to our overall immune system's health.

Probiotics can be found in dairy products like yogurt, kefir, sauerkraut, kimchi, miso, and kombucha.

Most studies show that between 1-10 billion CFU (colony forming units) is sufficient to help support your microbiome.

Oregano Oil

Oregano oil contains a substance called carvacrol which has been proven to have strong antioxidant properties and is excellent at fighting viruses and bacteria. Oregano oil has been said to help reduce sore throats and improve respiratory function in those suffering from the common cold and flu.

Oregano oil can be taken orally in a capsule or as a tincture. It can also be inhaled by putting a few drops of it in a diffuser.

No specific daily dose has been established for oregano oil, so taking the recommended dosage or seeking your medical or naturopathic doctor's advice.

Elderberry

Elderberry has gained popularity recently due to its immune-boosting properties and helping people recover from the Covid-19 virus. While it has been used for centuries for its healing properties, its use during this pandemic has seen and increased its demand. The elderberry is full of vitamins, minerals, and antioxidants that pack a powerful punch when it comes to fighting cold and flu viruses and some bacteria. Elderberry is also shown to have cardiovascular healing properties, which may help fight cancer and may even assist in combating depression.

Elderberry can be found in capsule or tincture form, or the berries can be cooked and eaten or made into a juice or jam.

It is advisable to follow the product label to determine the right amount of elderberry for you.

It is very important to note that you should speak to your pharmacist or healthcare provider to ensure that the product you are taking is right for you before taking any vitamins, minerals, or other supplements. Even natural supplements can have serious interactions with each other or with other medications that you may be on.

Sources

- https://ods.od.nih.gov/factsheets/Omega3FattyAcids-Health
- https://www.healthline.com/nutrition/echinacea
- https://www.healthline.com/health/oregano-oil-for-cold
- www.webbernaturals.com
- www.livescience.com/34693-superfoods.html
- https://askthescientists.com/vitamin-d-immunity/
- www.healthline.com/nutrition/10-foods-high-in-magnesium

Chapter Four
Body's in Motion, Will Stay in Motion

You may have heard the adage, "when you rest, you rust!" This is certainly true in the case of a car or a piece of machinery. If we leave it sitting there unused, its parts which are often made of iron will rust. The same rule applies to our bodies and our mind. In order to stay healthy, pain-free, and as young as possible, we need to keep moving and keep active.

The benefits of exercise are far-reaching. Exercise strengthens your cardiovascular system and thus reduces your risk of heart attack or stroke. Regular exercise builds muscle tissue that strengthens our physical body, improves stamina, boosts your metabolism, and improves brain function by increasing blood flow and oxygen to the brain. Daily exercise will increase your tolerance of pain, improve your balance, keep your weight in check, and keep you more engaged in your life and daily activities.

Beyond all of these benefits, regular exercise is also essential for keeping your immune system functioning efficiently.

Why is exercise important for my immune health?

There are so many different reasons that a daily physical exercise regime will boost your immunity and keep you better protected against illness and disease.

- **Exercise improves your sleep -** One of the great benefits of exercising is an improved quality of sleep. When our bodies are active throughout the day, it becomes much easier for us to fall asleep at night. A good night's rest is a vital part of allowing all of our important systems to regenerate and strengthen themselves, including our immune system.

- **Exercise reduces stress -** Stress is extremely hazardous to our health overall. Chronic stress puts our bodies into a constant state of "fight or flight, increasing stress hormones like cortisol and decreasing our immune system's ability to function and fight off disease. Exercise has been proven to reduce the effects of stress and gives us the ability to better deal with stressors that come up in our lives in the future.

- **Exercise boosts your mood -** When you exercise, your body produces endorphins and other chemicals that boost your mood. These effects can be long-lasting, lingering long after our exercise session is complete. A higher level of mood-boosting chemicals within your body is better for your body and your immune system overall, but being in a better mood also means that you will be better equipped to take care of yourself. We will also be more inclined to make better food choices that will boost our gut health and provide our bodies with the nutrition it needs to thrive.

- **Exercise reduces body weight -** This is not a secret! Being physically active builds muscle and burns fat, keeping our body weight in check. When we excess body fat, our bodies, and internal systems are under a constant state of inflammation. This inflammation causes our immune system to malfunction, increasing our risk of contracting a debilitating disease.

- An increased body mass also causes our cells to become more resistant to insulin, leading to an excess of glucose in the blood that cannot be properly taken up by our cells and used for energy as it is meant to be. If our bodies' cells aren't being provided with the energy they need to function and regenerate properly, they won't be able to fight off infection properly either.

Excess body fat also places an enormous strain on the organs of the body. These organs become surrounded by fatty tissue making it harder for them to work efficiently. Excess weight adversely affects all of the processes that take place within us. Our heart, lungs, kidney, liver, and even our brain will be affected by the fat surrounding them, having a detrimental effect on how they function, resulting in more illness and disease instances.

Finally, being overweight is often a sign of a poor diet. Suppose we aren't feeding ourselves with a wholesome, nutritious diet that is low in refined sugars, processed foods, and saturated fats. In that case, our microbiome will be out of balance, and our immune system will become impaired.

- **Exercise promotes good digestion** - While studies are still being conducted to find out exactly how it has been shown that people who exercise regularly have a more diverse and healthier microbiome than people who do not. It also promotes blood flow to the stomach, small and large intestines, which aids in digestion and moves waste through the system, and thus decreasing the chances of you becoming constipated.

- **Exercise makes you sweat** - Most of us think of sweating as just our body's way of regulating our temperature, but sweating does so much more. When we sweat, our body also flushes out toxins and certain heavy metals. While the liver and kidney are the primary organs of the body responsible for cleansing and removing toxins, sweating can assist with this as well.

- **Exercise reduces blood glucose levels** - When you exercise, your body needs fuel, and the fastest and easiest way for it to get the fuel it needs is by using up the glucose found in your blood. Also, a regular exercise regime helps to decrease insulin resistance and allows your body to use both insulin and, therefore, glucose more effectively.

- **Exercise helps fight bacteria** - Studies have shown that exercise can help to flush bacteria out of the lungs, which can decrease the chances of you catching a cold or other respiratory infection. When you exercise, your body temperature rises, which may help kill off any inside (similar to getting a fever).

- **Exercise helps the lymphatic system** - Our lymphatic system carries a fluid called lymph throughout our bodies, helping to shuttle nutrients. Unlike the cardiovascular system, which uses the heart to pump blood through the body, the lymphatic system doesn't have a pump. It relies on your body's movement to move the lymph fluid. Regular exercise keeps this fluid moving as it should.

How can exercise help with stress relief?

We all know that stress is extremely bad for our bodies. When we are under constant, chronic stress, our bodies go into survival mode. At our core level, our bodies are unable to distinguish between being attacked or being stressed out about our lives, our finances, and our jobs. The internal stress reaction is the same for both, and when we experience this stress for extended periods of time, our bodies begin to focus solely on survival. They pump out chemicals to help us deal with this stress instead of focusing on fighting viruses and keeping us healthy.

Exercise, especially moderate exercise that you enjoy, done three to five times per week, is an excellent way to combat the effects of stress.

- It produces endorphins and other feel-good hormones that boost our mood and decrease feelings of depression and anxiety.

- It helps to reduce our weight, causing an overall decrease in our blood pressure and heart rate.

- It allows us to focus on our breathing, essentially acting as a form of meditation that helps calm both our bodies and minds.

- It's distracting! It's hard to focus on the things in our lives that stress us out when we are focused on doing something physical.

- It gives you energy and allows you to get more done throughout your day.

- It helps to provide mental clarity and reduce brain fog which can help you deal more efficiently with stressful issues as they arise throughout your day.

- It helps you sleep better at night, giving both your body and mind a chance to rest and regenerate.

- It helps to loosen up your body and relieves tension in your muscles, helping you to feel more relaxed.

- It improves your confidence levels and your body image.

When we take steps to reduce the stress in our lives through regular exercise, we can reap the benefits of a healthier body and a stronger mind. Less stress also means that we have an immune system that is better equipped to fight sickness and disease.

How much exercise do I need each day?

The type and amount of exercise that you need each day completely depends on your personal circumstances. Someone looking to lose weight will require more exercise than someone looking to maintain their body weight. Similarly, someone looking to gain muscle and tone their body will require more weight-bearing exercises than someone looking to improve their cardiovascular health.

As a general rule, however, twenty to thirty minutes of moderate exercise, three to five times per week, should provide you with all of the benefits that exercise has to offer on both your entire wellness and the health of your immune system.

To start, choose an exercise that you enjoy and gradually start incorporating it into your daily routine. Start slow, and work your way up to a pace and duration that is comfortable for you. The more you do it, the easier it will be!

Examples of exercises to keep me active and healthy

When people hear the term "exercise," they often think of hours of extreme physical exertion or lifting extremely heavy amounts of weight at the gym. While this may work for the professionals, excess physical exercise may actually be harmful for the average person, leading to increased bodily stress levels, increased incidence of physical injury, and an overall decline in immune function.

The average person should get between twenty minutes and one hour of moderate physical activity, three to five days a week. When choosing an activity, think of something that you like to do and try to make it as much fun as possible. Listen to music or a podcast, exercise while watching your favorite TV show, or get a group of friends together to work out together. The more you enjoy the activity you are doing, the more likely you will be to keep it up and make it a part of your weekly routine.

Here are some fun ways to add physical activity to your life:

- Go for a walk outside.
- Try yoga
- Have a dance party around your house
- Try a workout video
- Join a Tai Chi class
- Go swimming
- Gather your friends for a sports game or join a local team
- Spend time gardening

- Take the stairs
- Park at the back of the parking lot

Why is mental exercise important?

Most of the time, when we think of exercise, we think of keeping our bodies fit and in shape, but keeping our minds exercised is just as important. When we exercise our mind, we increase the amount of gray matter it contains, essentially making us smarter and allowing our brain to function better. When our brain is functioning optimally, so will the rest of our body, including our immune system.

Here are some excellent exercises to try to strengthen your mind:

- Reading
- Word games
- Puzzles
- Riddles
- Learn a new language
- Play a computer or board game
- Practice memory exercises
- Learn to cook
- Play cards

We have always known that both physical and mental exercise is good for our body, but now we know that it is an essential part of our immune health. Staying fit and active will allow us to be stronger, have more energy, sleep better and fight off illness and disease more effectively.

Next, we will look at the hazards of prescription drugs, how they affect our health, and the detrimental effects they have on our immune system.

Sources

- https://www.sciencedaily.com/releases/2020/03/200331162314.htm
- www.pubmed.ncbi.nlm.nih.gov/15678717/
- https://pubmed.ncbi.nlm.nih.gov/11115789/
- https://medlineplus.gov/ency/article/007165.htm
- https://www.health.harvard.edu/mind-and-mood/more-evidence-that-exercise-can-boost-mood
- https://universityhealthnews.com/daily/digestive-health/the-benefits-of-exercise-for-digestive-health/

Chapter Five
Live A Drug-Free Life

When we hear about the danger of taking drugs, our minds immediately turn to drugs like Cocaine, Heroin, and Methamphetamine. From childhood, we have been warned not to take these drugs. Yet, we are hardly ever told about the detrimental effects that prescription drugs can have on our health. We are taught from an early age to trust our doctors and to take, without question, whatever medication that they prescribe for us.

While it's true that many medical advancements have extended our lifespan and increased our quality of life, many other medications that are available on the market come with a whole list of side effects. In contrast, many others often don't treat the actual disease but instead alleviate one or more of the symptoms.

When a doctor prescribes a medication for you to take, he or she does so knowing that the medication may cause you harm. They know that there is the potential for side effects, drug interactions, or drug allergies. However, they must decide if the benefits of taking the medication outweigh the risk of you having an adverse reaction to it. In my opinion, other than in a life or death situation, taking such medication should never be the first option.

As we have learned in previous chapters, boosting our immune system by eating healthy and embracing a physical lifestyle is one of the best ways to prevent disease and to fight off any future illness that we may encounter. While prescription drugs may have their time and place for treating certain conditions, living a drug-free life is one of the best ways to keep your immune system strong and healthy for years to come.

Why are pharmaceuticals bad for you?

Almost all medications are bad for you, in one way or another. Even the Food and Drug Administration (FDA), which is the government agency responsible for approving all pharmaceutical drugs prescribed by doctors, acknowledges this. A pharmaceutical drug gets FDA approval when the benefits of taking it outweigh the inherent side effects associated with it.

- **A medication may cause side effects** - When taking the medication to treat one thing, you may end up contracting a whole host of other medical problems. Some common side effects of taking such medications include constipation, nausea, diarrhea, drowsiness, insomnia, skin problems, mood changes, or changes in blood pressure, to name a few. Side effects are usually well known and well documented.

- The drug companies, by law, have to tell you about the side effects of their drugs in their television commercials that flood our airways and magazines.

  In my opinion, drug companies should not be allowed to promote their products to the general public. This is because the public does not have the necessary medical training to know whether a particular drug is appropriate for treating their medical condition. By advertising on television, drug companies are bypassing the medical professionals who have been trained to decide whether or not a particular drug should be prescribed to their patient or not. Thus, the drug companies become the defacto doctors to the general public. The reason why they are doing this is obvious. Pharmaceutical companies want to maximize their profits by persuading as many people as possible to buy their drugs.

What's worse is that by being allowed to advertise their drugs on television, the drug companies are effectively recruiting an army of unpaid sales representatives to sell their products to as many people as they can. Thus, they make the public the agents of their destruction because they are selling these drugs to themselves.

A medication may cause an adverse reaction - As mentioned earlier, there are many side effects associated with pharmaceutical drugs. Drug dependence, organ damage or failure, carcinogenic effects, or seizures are all examples of adverse drug reactions.

Just watch one of the many drug commercials that we are forced to watch each day and listen to the myriad of side effects associated with them.

I believe that the FDA has done the public a huge disservice by allowing drug companies to advertise their products on television. Why would the FDA allow drug companies to sell their products directly to the general public, knowing that they are not qualified to decide whether or not a particular drug should be prescribed to treat a disease that they have? They are doing this because there is an unholy alliance between the FDA and big pharma.

The more severe side effects associated with these drugs often result in the patient being prescribed additional drugs to counteract them. As already stated, when a person is taking two or more prescription drugs, they increase their risk of having an adverse reaction to them.

- **A medication may cause a drug interaction** - When a person takes multiple prescription drugs, they are at increased risk of experiencing side effects from taking one or more of such drugs. This is because one drug's chemical interaction with another drug has caused such a side effect to occur. Prescribing multiple drugs is also problematic because one drug may reduce the efficacy of another drug. This means that the patient is no longer deriving the full benefit of taking such a medication. This means that the patient will have to take an increased dosage of the drug to increase its efficacy. However, doing this increases the chance that the patient will experience one or more of the serious side effects associated with taking that drug.

- **A medication may cause a drug allergy** - A drug allergy is an adverse reaction of your immune system to a pharmaceutical drug. The drug could either be prescription or non-prescription. Both are capable of inducing a drug allergy. It should also be noted that people can also have an allergic reaction to herbal remedies and supplements too. However, a drug allergy is more likely to occur as a result of taking a pharmaceutical drug. Mild allergic reactions include minor skin irritations, rashes, and hives. Major allergic reactions are called anaphylactic reactions and are life-threatening. A person experiencing anaphylaxis would experience severe swelling of the face, lips, and throat and difficulty breathing. Some drugs that are well-known for causing these reactions include penicillin's, cephalosporins, NSAID's, Sulfa drugs, IV contrast dyes, and local anesthetics.

While all of these may seem like enough reasons to avoid taking prescription drugs, we have another very important reason that regular prescription drugs are bad for you. That is, they have an extremely harmful effect on our immune system.

Our immune system's proper functioning relies on a very delicate balance of several different things. Our microbiome, the nutrients we receive, our hormones, and our bodies' overall wellbeing as a whole. The purpose of a medication is to treat the symptoms of a disease or disorder.

For example, we may be prescribed a proton pump inhibitor (also known as a PPI) to help reduce the amount of acid our stomachs produce to minimize the symptoms of heartburn and acid reflux. While this therapy is often very successful in treating heartburn, the effects of long-term use can be very harmful to the body. Acid Reflux disease is caused by an imbalance in the microbiome in our gut due to bad eating habits. Instead of addressing the cause of the disease by treating it at its root, we take the medication that essentially acts as a band-aid for the symptoms only. We may feel better, but our microbiome is now completely out of balance from continued consumption of unhealthy foods plus the use of PPI medication which is reducing the normal flow of acid to our stomach. This can also lead to malnourishment as our food will no longer be broken down and properly absorbed into the body. This could lead to a host of other health problems that could require the patient to take additional prescription drugs. It's like a bad game of dominoes; one relatively simple problem has now led to an entire chain reaction that has affected the entire body in so many different ways.

Some medications may alter our mood, which in turn can alter our appetites, causing us to lose it completely or promoting cravings for unhealthy foods. This can lead to malnourishment or unhealthy gut flora.

Other medications may cause drowsiness or an overall feeling of exhaustion. This can lead to inactivity and eventually weight gain, which can both factors that can have a negative impact on the immune system.

What's worse is that some prescription drugs actually suppress the immune system on purpose (immunosuppressant medications), wearing down the body's defense mechanism and making it extremely easy to get sick.

As you can see, different medications may have a different way of affecting the immune system, but the end result is almost always the same. In one way or another, adding unnatural chemicals to the body to deal with symptoms of a bigger problem can often end up making you sicker in the long run.

The pharmaceutical testing and approval process

You may be wondering how prescription drugs could be so bad for us. After all, they go through a rigorous testing process that ensures they are completely safe, right?

Wrong!

While pharmaceutical drugs are tested, the results of these tests are only so valuable. First, as we mentioned before, these drugs are allowed to be put onto the market and sold to the public with the full knowledge that they can cause potential harm. As we talked about previously, as long as the FDA feels that the benefits of taking the medication outweigh the many risks involved, the medication will be approved. This means that even though there are significant potential risks involved, the drug will still be sold to the public.

The FDA also allows for a fast-track process, a breakthrough therapy process, and a priority review for new medications that are still being developed. If these drugs meet certain criteria, their testing phase is expedited, and they can be released to the general public before all of their clinical trials are completed. This means that the long-term effects of the medications are unknown.

From the very creation of a new drug, through the development process and all of the studies and clinical trials, a new medication may be brought to market in as little as five to seven years. Even though the drug approval process takes several years, it often fails to discover harmful and even fatal side effects that can result from its use. As proof of this, take a quick look at the news or on Google and see just how many drugs have been taken off the market because new information has shown that they are no longer safe for people to take. Many people have lost their lives because the medications they believed would cure or treat their illness were not sufficiently tested. It could also be because they were not tested for a long enough time so that the scientists that developed them could fully understand the hazards and health consequences they could cause.

Stay away from antibiotics!

In 1928, Professor Alexander Fleming discovered penicillin and changed the world. Illnesses that people would previously die from now became a simple fix. All you had to do was take a few pills, and you'd be fine. This breakthrough discovery has changed the way we live and has greatly increased our lifespan and quality of life.

While it is true to say that antibiotics have greatly improved our quality of life, it needs to be said that antibiotics have also endangered our lives too.

Let's first take a look at bacterial resistance. Bacterial resistance occurs when antibiotics are overused, which creates a serious problem. When we take antibiotics too often or for the wrong reasons or start a course but don't complete the entire prescription as directed by the doctor, the bacteria will not be completely eradicated from our body. It begins to mutate, becoming stronger, and the antibiotic becomes useless. We now have a drug-resistant bacteria that could potentially be spread around from person to person and create a major health crisis. This means that scientists have to find stronger antibiotics to kill these superbugs. The fear is that eventually, one of these superbugs will resist all attempts to kill it.

It is extremely important that if you or anyone in your house takes antibiotics, it is only extremely important that they are being taken to eliminate serious bacterial infection (not a viral infection) and that the entire course of antibiotics is completed.

Antibiotics are also extremely dangerous to our immune system. As we know, our body produces important bacteria that are vital for our good health, and this bacterium is directly responsible for the development and maintenance of our white blood cells. Antibiotics not only kill off the bad bacteria that we have in our body but also kill off the good bacteria too. This means that with fewer good bacteria, our white blood cells will suffer, and our immunity to sickness and diseases will be compromised. We will be ill equipped to fight future infections. We may also experience an overgrowth of other substances, such as yeast, leading to fungal infections.

We know that our microbiome's delicate balance is very important for maintaining a good and healthy immune system, and taking antibiotics is one surefire way to disrupt this balance.

Before taking antibiotics, talk to your healthcare provider first. Ask the following questions to determine what the best course of action is:

- Am I suffering from a viral or bacterial infection?

- How serious is my infection?

- Is there a natural treatment that I can try first?

- What natural remedies could help treat my symptoms?

If you are suffering from a viral infection, there is nothing that an antibiotic will be able to do for you. Therefore, taking natural remedies to help your symptoms will be the best course of action. If you get a common bacterial infection, a herbal remedy will treat your symptoms and enable your body's Immune system to deal with it. If after a few days the infection has gotten worse, please seek immediate medical care.

Take preventative measures

One of the best ways to ensure that you don't need to take prescription drugs in the first place is to keep your immune system strong and healthy. One of the best ways to do this is to:

- Eat a clean and healthy diet filled with plenty of whole foods, fruits, vegetables, nuts, and seeds. Remember that the more colorful your diet and the less processed the foods you eat, the healthier and more nutritious they are. Try to keep your grocery shopping to the grocery store's outside aisles and ensure that all of your meals are wholesome and nutrient-dense.

- Take a probiotic every day. Probiotics will help to keep your gut flora healthy and balanced and will promote a strong immune system.

- Take immune-boosting supplements like the ones we spoke about in the chapter on supplements. There are a wide variety of different immune-boosting herbal products that can give your immune system the extra help that it needs, such as vitamin C, zinc, oregano oil, elderberry, and echinacea.

- Wash your hands often, especially before eating, to remove any viruses or bacteria that you may have inadvertently come in contact with during your regular, daily activities.

What should I do if I get sick?

If you find yourself not feeling well, don't panic. Despite all of our best efforts to stay healthy, sometimes we still get sick

When that happens, you should:

- **Contact your naturopath or healthcare provider** - They will be able to give you the best possible advice on how to treat your symptoms, boost your immunity against what has made you sick, and fight off whatever ailment that has made you sick.

- **Keep taking your supplements** - Make sure that you are still taking your daily probiotics and any other supplements that you usually take. Your body relies on all of these things to help keep your immune system strong while under attack.

- **Continue to eat a healthy diet** - While we often don't feel like eating when we are unwell, our bodies need the strength and nutrition that a healthy diet will provide. Thus it is of paramount importance to eat healthy foods because they will empower your Immune system to fight off the sickness that has caused you to become unwell. Also, make sure that you are staying well hydrated. Drinking plenty of nonsugary drinks will help your body flush out the virus or bacterium that has made you sick.

- **Try natural remedies** - Natural remedies like ginger and garlic have bacterial fighting properties and can help your body fight off any infection much faster. Echinacea can help decrease the severity of your illness. Also, adding honey and lemon to your tea will help keep you hydrated and soothe the symptoms of a sore throat or cough and help fight off infection as well.

Recreational drugs and your immune system

While taking prescription drugs can have a detrimental effect on your immunity, the hazards of taking street recreational drugs like heroin and cocaine can have an even more detrimental effect it. Many people only use street drugs occasionally, and since they don't indulge every day, they feel they are doing minimal harm to themselves by taking them. This is simply not true! Street drugs are very strong, and the whole purpose of taking them is to achieve a feeling of euphoria. They affect vital bodily functions that are necessary for good immunity and, therefore, good health.

What do recreational drugs do to your immune system?

While studies are still being done on the effects of recreational drugs and how they affect the immune system, a few things are clear. First, the use of recreational drugs increases your exposure to microbial contaminants. Sharing joints or paraphernalia along with the use of needles increases your chances of being exposed to pathogens and therefore increases your chances of getting sick.

Certain drugs, especially opioids, are also thought to attach to receptors on immune cells, which directly results in the suppression of a person's immune system and the immune response. This means that if you do become infected with a virus or bacteria, your immune system will be weakened, and you won't be able to fight it off as efficiently.

Finally, when you are high on street drugs, you most likely aren't giving your full consideration to how you are fueling your body. You may make unhealthy food choices or forget to stay hydrated, weakening your body. Drugs are also very addictive, and once you get hooked, your main concern won't be on making healthy choices and boosting your immunity. Your only focus will be on getting your next hit. This usually leads to a downward spiral of a person's overall health and wellbeing.

The hazards of smoking on your immunity

Thankfully the number of smokers in our society is gradually decreasing. What was once a popular habit is now generally frowned upon, and more and more people are proudly calling themselves quitters. While this may be true, there are still a significant number of people who partake in this habit, and it can be extremely detrimental to your immune system.

Smoking directly affects many of your white blood cells (called T-cells) that are specifically responsible for fighting infection. They decrease the cell's ability to fight, weaken the immune system and even have cytotoxic effects - killing off otherwise healthy cells. Smoking causes inflammation in the body (especially in the lungs), making your body more susceptible to infection. Cigarettes are also known to be carcinogenic, causing cell mutations and promoting cancer growth.

The hazards of alcohol on your immune system

Is alcohol bad for you? Yes and no. Including a very small amount of alcohol, specifically red wine, into your diet can actually help your immune system. Red wine is known to contain immune-boosting polyphenols, and when consumed responsibly and in moderation, can actually help boost your immunity.

On the other hand, drinking other types of alcoholic beverages like beer, whiskey or vodka, or consuming alcohol in excess can significantly affect your immune system and make you more susceptible to illness and disease.

Wine coolers, hard lemonade, shandy, and similar alcoholic beverages contain very high amounts of sugar, which, as we have already learned, is very bad for your gut health and can cause an imbalance in your body's microbiome.

Drinking alcohol can also lead to dehydration. It is a diuretic and pushes fluid from the body. Staying hydrated is extremely important for our immune system's health, and drinking alcohol, especially in excess, can deplete our body's fluid levels.

Alcohol, especially when consumed in excess, can affect immune cells, inhibiting their ability to function properly. It also affects the liver, which is the main organ in our body that is responsible for filtering toxins out of our body. If the liver doesn't function properly, our bodies can become filled with toxins, quickly leading to illness and disease.

Finally, if all of these other reasons weren't enough to convince you of the hazards of drinking, alcohol can also be extremely addictive and can impair your judgment. When you are impaired, you will make poor lifestyle choices and poor nutritional choices too. We have already discussed how not eating and drinking healthy things will negatively impact your health.

Sources

- https://www.fda.gov/drugs/information-consumers-and-patients-drugs/think-it-through-managing-benefits-and-risks-medicines
- https://www.verywellhealth.com/drug-allergy-83059
- https://pubmed.ncbi.nlm.nih.gov/26619012/
- https://www.fda.gov/drugs/development-approval-process-drugs
- https://www.healthline.com/health-news/antibiotics-hurt-your-health-unless-you-have-an-infection#Antibiotics-damage-the-ability-of-our-white-blood-cells
- https://www.ncbi.nlm.nih.gov/pmc/articles/PMC153143/
- https://www.ncbi.nlm.nih.gov/pmc/articles/PMC5352117/

Chapter Six
The Truth About Vaccines

Did you know that vaccines have been around for thousands of years? In 1000 A.D., there are accounts of early Chinese practitioners scraping the fluid from smallpox sores into the arms of uninfected people in an attempt to protect them from the deadly disease. Throughout the centuries, doctors and scientists have continued to research ways to protect against certain viruses and diseases and have been successful, on many counts, in eradicating illnesses that were once extremely prevalent and deadly.

Louis Pasteur is perhaps one of the best known names in early vaccine history and discovered the vaccine for anthrax poisoning and rabies. As a result of his work and discoveries, other scientists became involved in the search for new vaccines against viruses, bacteria, and venom. By 1980, smallpox had been completely eradicated, and other diseases like polio had been greatly decreased.

What is a vaccine?

A vaccine can be administered either through injection, orally as a suspension or in pill form, or as a nasal spray and contains either a very small part of the virus or bacteria or contains active antibodies of the disease from an animal or human donor. Once administered, the vaccine will trigger a response in your body which will cause antibodies to be produced by the B-cells. These cells go to work attacking the vaccine and essentially store the information about the pathogen in the cell memory, ensuring that if your body ever comes into contact with it again, it is immediately recognized as an intruder and fought off.

Let's take a quick look at some of the different types of vaccine technology:

- **Attenuated Vaccines -** An attenuated vaccine uses a very small amount of the live virus or bacteria to produce an immune response in the body. The measles, mumps, rubella, shingles, and yellow fever vaccines are all examples of attenuated vaccines.

- **Inactivated Vaccines -** This type of vaccine uses a dead version of the germ to produce immunity in the body and is usually weaker than the attenuated types. Due to this fact, many doses (boosters) are often required to build up a strong level of immunity. Examples of inactivated vaccines include Hepatitis A, rabies, and polio.

- **Subunit Vaccine or Recombinant DNA -** Subunit vaccines use only a very small part of the pathogen, such as a protein molecule, a piece of its cell casing, or a part of its DNA, to cause the body to produce an immune response that is specific to identifying only that one, specific pathogen. This type of vaccine is usually considered safer than some of the other varieties because the small part of the germ contained in the vaccine cannot infect the system. Therefore, it can be used on people who have weak immune systems. Hepatitis A, HPV, pneumonia, and meningitis vaccines are all examples that use this type of technology. These vaccines usually require booster shots to keep up the body's immunity.

- **Messenger RNA Vaccines -** This is one of the newest forms of vaccine technology and is currently being used for most of the COVID-19 vaccinations. Instead of using a piece of the pathogen that we are seeking immunity from, mRNA vaccines are like messengers that directly "speak" to our immune cells and teach them how to fight off a specific germ. While this is a complicated technology, researchers have been studying it for several years and have also been considered for use as a cancer treatment.

Are vaccines safe?

There is currently a huge, world-wide debate about whether vaccines are safe or not. The evidence supporting both sides of this debate is quite compelling. Vaccines have greatly improved our way of life by eradicating many diseases and illnesses that once plagued our society. Still, recent studies have shown that they can cause many illnesses of their own. Let's take a look at both sides of the vaccine debate, as this will help us decide whether or not we should get vaccinated or have our children vaccinated against a particular virus.

Pros to getting Vaccinated

- Vaccines for viruses are very important because viruses do not react to antibiotics. If you get sick with a virus, there is no cure in many cases, and they are very difficult to treat.

- Vaccines play an important role in impoverished countries where there is a lack of medical care. People who get vaccinated are less likely to get sick with certain illnesses and therefore won't suffer the often deadly symptoms that these illnesses cause.

- Vaccines are important if you don't have access to a doctor or don't have the funds to get proper medical treatment. Preventing an illness is much less expensive than having to treat one.

- Many vaccines have been on the market for decades and have been administered to thousands of people. They have also undergone years of research and testing and have been deemed safe for use.

- Getting vaccinated helps protect others from getting sick, keeping your friends, family, and coworkers safe.

- Vaccines can help save you money by decreasing the amount of sick time that you miss from work.

Cons to getting vaccinated

- Vaccinations can be painful, can cause fevers, and in rare cases may cause febrile seizures.

- In rare cases, vaccines may cause a severe allergic reaction.

- In other cases, when a live vaccine is used, it may cause you to become sick with the very disease that it is meant to prevent you from contracting.

- Even after getting vaccinated, there is still a chance that the vaccine will not work, meaning that you may get the disease that it was given to you to prevent.

- Some vaccines only protect against certain strains of a virus (for example, the flu or the current corona-virus). Therefore, if you get infected with another strain, then the vaccine you have taken won't protect you.

- Many vaccines are mandatory, and proof of this must be provided in order for you to travel to certain countries or in order for your children to attend school. This takes away your right to decide what you want or don't want to put into your or your children's bodies.

- Most vaccines are not 100% effective. Most vaccines are between 50% - 75% effective in protecting against the intended disease.

- Some vaccines can contain harmful ingredients, such as mercury.

- Some studies have shown that if a person has been vaccinated against a certain virus and is later exposed to that virus, their immune response to that virus is much stronger and more aggressive. This puts a strain on the overall immune system, causing it to weaken.

- Some vaccines have been linked to causing other diseases such as autism, Guillain-Barre syndrome, rheumatoid arthritis, and multiple sclerosis.

The decision to get vaccinated or to get your children vaccinated should be yours and yours alone to make. Accept that the government should not be mandating you to do so in the case of an outbreak of a very deadly and very virulent virus. As you can see, there are many pros and cons and the decision isn't an easy one. Arming yourself with a wide range of unbiased information should help make the decision easier and more educated.

The link between vaccines and other diseases

While studies have been inconclusive, many researchers have found a direct link between getting vaccinated and certain diseases. Some of the most common diseases that have been associated with vaccinations include:

- **Guillain-Barre syndrome -** This disease is a neurological disorder that occurs when your immune system begins attacking your nervous system, causing weakness, tingling, and eventually paralysis. Many studies have shown that after a yearly flu vaccine program, the incidence of this syndrome increases.

- **Arthritis -** Arthritis is a disease of the joints in the body and causes pain and inflammation. Like the rubella vaccine, certain vaccinations have shown an increase in joint problems, including arthritis.

- **Multiple Sclerosis -** This autoimmune disease has been linked to vaccinations for HPV and hepatitis B. Studies have shown that people that have been given these vaccinations are at an increased risk for M.S. However, it remains unclear if these vaccines directly cause the disease or activate the disease in people who were previously unaware that they had it.

- **Autism** - This developmental disorder has been associated with the MMR vaccine. While some studies have shown that there is no link between getting vaccinated and developing the disorder, the research still seems to be ongoing. Other studies have shown that there may be a link between the mercury contained in the MMR vaccine and autism. Studies have shown that the mercury content in vaccines can cause mental disorders like autism and cerebral palsy.

- While there is still a lot to be learned and studied about the potential for vaccinations to lead to long-term health complications, studies have shown that there are many links that may be cause for serious concern.

- While vaccines play an important role in eradicating disease, determining whether a vaccine is the right choice for you and your family can be a very personal decision. When deciding whether or not to get vaccinated or to vaccinate your children, you should consider all of the different factors relating to your current health. You should also check out all available information on the safety and effectiveness of the vaccine too. It's important that you make an educated decision, weighing both the benefits and the potential hazards and that you do what is right for you.

Sources

- https://www.historyofvaccines.org/timeline#EVT_1
- https://www.vaccines.gov/basics/types
- https://www.healthline.com/health/vaccinations/opposition

- https://www.cdc.gov/flu/prevent/guillainbarre.htm
- https://www.ncbi.nlm.nih.gov/books/NBK234372/
- https://pubmed.ncbi.nlm.nih.gov/25329096/

Chapter Seven
Stress, the Silent Killer

We all know how it feels to be under stress. In the society that we live in, it's a common, everyday occurrence. We wake up in the morning, rush off to work, fight our way through crowded streets and then push our way through tight deadlines. We do the same thing on the way home and then run out to practice, only to find ourselves completely exhausted and burnt out at the end of the day.

If this sounds all too familiar, you are not alone. The majority of people in our society suffer from stress on a daily basis, and this stress is leading to bigger and more severe health consequences. It takes a toll on our mental wellbeing and physical health, leading to more anxiety and depression and an overall weakened immune system.

However, learning to deal with this stress can be easy and can be something that we implement into our daily routines. By taking the time to learn some simple techniques, we can not only improve our mood, but we can also bolster up our immune systems and ensure that we live the longest, healthiest life possible.

Let's take a deep dive into the two different types of stress and how they affect us.

The different types of stress

There are two very different types of stress that can affect us, and they each have a different effect on our body. The stress response is specifically designed to keep us alive, but it can actually cause us a great deal of harm when it malfunctions due to extreme and long-lasting stress.

Acute stress occurs when we face an immediate stressful situation that threatens our survival, like an animal attack or an imminent car accident. This type of stress comes on very quickly and sends our bodies into overdrive. An immediate trigger reaction, called the fight or flight response, ensues. This response causes our bodies to produce hormones like corticotropin and cortisol, our blood pressure and heart rate speed up, we begin to sweat, we produce more glycogen to use as fuel, and the adrenal glands begin pumping out adrenaline. Our blood vessels constrict, our pupils dilate, and the bronchi in our lungs dilate as well to allow as much oxygen in as possible. Our bodies are on high alert, ready to react and either run away or stay and fight for survival.

This fight or flight response is what has allowed the human race to overcome danger and stay alive through life-threatening situations since the dawn of time. It gives us the focus, strength, and quick reaction time that we need to immediately think through a problem and react to the best possible chance of surviving the situation.

Chronic Stress - Chronic stress occurs when we find ourselves suffering from stressful situations for an extended period of time. Factors like our job, our family life, and our finances can play a strong role in the amount of stress that we feel, and if this stress isn't handled properly and is allowed to take over, we can begin to suffer the effects of chronic stress.

Like acute stress, when the body is under chronic, long-term stress, it undergoes the fight or flight response. The only difference is that the body doesn't have time to relax again in between. When we become overwhelmed by stress, our body pumps out hormones and adrenaline in anticipation of an imminent threat. This constant state of stress wears down our body, never giving it the chance to rest and relax, and has an extremely detrimental effect on all of our bodily functions, including our immune system.

The adverse effect of stress on the immune system

One of the biggest hazards to your immune system when you are under chronic, long-term stress is the constant release of the stress hormone cortisol. This hormone is extremely important for the fight or flight response to work properly and can save your life in a dangerous situation. However, when dealing with chronic stress, cortisol can have some very detrimental effects on the body. One of the major hazards of this hormone is that it stops the production of lymphocytes which are the body's main defense against infection. Your immune system becomes suppressed, meaning that you will be much more susceptible to infection and have the potential to suffer longer and more severe illnesses since your body will have a harder time fighting pathogens off.

This constant state of being in the fight or flight response can also cause:

- **Adrenal Fatigue** - When your body is under stress for a long period of time, your adrenal glands become taxed. They have been pumping out cortisol for so long that they can no longer continue to produce the usual amounts of both cortisol and the other hormones that they are responsible for. This can cause symptoms such as extreme tiredness, food cravings, weight gain, insomnia, brain fog, and decreased libido.

- **High Blood Pressure** - The hormones that are released during stressful situations cause our blood pressure to rise. This is a natural reaction to acute stress; however, chronic stress, in our everyday lives, can lead to chronic high blood pressure, also known as hypertension.

- **Anxiety and Depression** - Chemicals in our body that are released due to stress, such as cortisol and adrenaline, can cause us to feel jittery and on edge. This is especially helpful in a life or death situation as it makes us alert and able to react quickly. However, during chronic stress, the constant release of these hormones and chemicals can cause us to feel anxious, depressed and can even bring on panic attacks.

- **Weight Gain** - The increased cortisol production that occurs when you are under constant, chronic stress causes your body to pull glucose out of its cells where it is usually stored. Your body does this in anticipation of the excess energy that it thinks you may need to either run or fight. Since you aren't in a life-threatening situation, eventually, your body will store this glucose again, and often it does this by creating fat stores. Chronic, increased cortisol production can lead to substantial weight gain, especially around the midsection.

- **Diabetes** - As we just mentioned, increased cortisol production leads to elevated glucose levels. If glucose levels stay elevated for a prolonged period of time, it can lead to metabolic disorders such as Type 2 diabetes.

- **Insomnia** - Many people find themselves suffering from insomnia. When we are presented with stressful situations all the time and aren't able to deal with them properly, it becomes hard to shut our minds off and calm our bodies down enough to be able to fall asleep and stay asleep at night.

If you are under chronic stress, it doesn't matter what your symptoms are. All symptoms of stress are detrimental to your body, mind, and overall wellbeing, no matter how minimal or severe the symptoms may be. If you experience any of these symptoms, they can snowball into other areas of your life. Chronic stress can cause things like brain fog, memory issues, poor eating habits, and lack of exercise, meaning that no matter how hard you try, you just won't be able to take care of yourself as well as you should. When you are under stress, your whole body, including your immune system, is stressed as well.

So what can you do about it? Let's take a look at some easy ways to deal with the stress in our lives.

5 Ways to combat stress

Learning to deal with the stress in our lives isn't always an easy task, but the harder we work at it, the less of an effect that stress will have on us. By being proactive and bringing about a sense of calm before stress can take over, we protect our bodies, minds, and especially our immune systems from becoming ill from the detrimental effects that stress can cause.

Here are just a few examples of methods that we can try to combat the stress in our lives and bring about a greater sense of peace and wellbeing.

1. Meditation

I'm sure you've heard the term meditation before, but have you ever given it a try? If you're like most of the population, you probably haven't, which means that you are missing out on so many amazing benefits! Not only can it help to combat stress and all of its symptoms, but it can make you better prepared to handle all of the stress that you may face in the future. It can help relax you, calm panic attacks and anxiety, reduce blood pressure, decrease insomnia, and help with mood, memory, and ability to focus. Plus, as an added bonus, it's easy, requires no investment, and can be done by anyone, anywhere!

What is meditation?

Despite what you may think, meditation isn't all about religious people in long white robes, sitting cross-legged on the ground with their eyes closed for hours and their hands in funny positions. Unfortunately, the media has presented us with this image, and it seems to have stuck. Many people now believe that meditation is only for monks or for spiritual people who have trained for years in an attempt to reach enlightenment. Because of this incorrect assumption, so many people are missing out on all of the benefits that meditation can provide.

So, what is meditation?

Meditation is the practice of focusing your mind, clearing your thoughts, and essentially slowing down. By working to keep your focus on one thing, you can keep your mind from continually racing and can slow your breathing, your heart rate, and your blood pressure, producing a calming effect throughout your body. At first, you may find it very difficult to focus on a single thing. However, with practice, you will be better able to stop racing thoughts and bring about concentration and clarity. Meditation can be done anytime, anywhere, and by anyone.

Types of Meditation

There are many different ways for us to practice meditation. It is also recommended that you try out different types of meditation to see which one works best for you.

Here are some of the most common types of meditation:

- **Breathing Meditation -** A breathing meditation is one of the easiest types of meditation to do. You can practice this type of meditation with your eyes open or closed and even try it while participating in other activities like driving or waiting in line at the grocery store. All you need to do is bring all of your attention to your breath. Focus on breathing in and breathing out. Feel the gentle rhythm of your breath and if other distracting thoughts or feelings come into your awareness, simply push them aside and bring your focus back to your breath.

- **Guided Meditation** - Guided meditations are especially beneficial for people who find it difficult to keep their concentration from wavering. A guided meditation is usually read by someone else, and it takes you on a journey. By providing detailed imagery for you to focus on, you will be able to push out stressful thoughts and focus only on the images suggested to you. There are excellent, free guided meditations for you to try on YouTube, social media, or on a meditation app.

- **Body Scan Meditation** - Body Scan Meditations are especially helpful in bringing about a strong mind/body connection. While they are a great way to calm the mind, they produce excellent relaxation effects on the body as well.

  To try this method, lay down, close your eyes and bring your focus to your feet, trying to physically relax every muscle. Next, move your attention to your calves, feel any sensations here, and make an effort to relax your calves muscles. Continue to move up your body, focusing on every area, relaxing any clenched muscles, and working towards complete relaxation. You can also find guided Body Scan Meditations, which may help those who find their mind wandering during this process.

  Body Scan Meditations are perfect to try in bed at night before going to sleep, and many people who do this find that they bring about a greater sense of relaxation and promote deeper and more restful sleep.

- **Music Meditation** - Many people don't realize that listening to their favorite music is also a type of meditation, but it is! Anything that clears our minds of negative thoughts and brings about focus and calm is a type of meditation. Try putting on your favorite tunes and sing along or put on a completely different type of music and pay attention to the rhythm, the individual instruments, and the words being sung. If stressful thoughts try to work their way into your mind, simply take a deep breath, push them out, and continue to focus on the music.

For this exercise to work well, try to choose uplifting or calming music that you like.

- **Walking Meditation** - Walking meditation is an excellent way to get your body up and moving while also working towards clearing your mind. Walking meditation is just like regular meditation, except it is done while you are up and walking around. Many people find it easier to clear their mind and focus while they are moving. Try to find one thing to focus your mind on, such as your breath, a mantra, or a song, and push out any stressful, intruding thoughts whenever they pop up.

- **Mantra Meditation** - A mantra is a word or phrase that you focus on during meditation. Using a mantra can be an excellent way to create a sense of calm and will be useful when faced with stressful situations. Choosing a mantra is easy; simply pick a word or phrase that resonates with you and repeat this word during your meditation or throughout your day if you find yourself feeling anxious. Mantras can be a very powerful tool for bringing about clarity, focus, and calm.

  Some mantras you could try are:

  "I am calm."

  "I am focused."

  "I feel amazing."

  "I am healthy."

- **Mala Meditation** - Malas are tools that have been used for centuries to assist with both meditation and prayer. They are a string of beads that help keep your focus and act as a timer while meditating. Each bead represents one cycle of breath or one mantra. When you have completed one round of the mala, your session is complete. Many people find that using a mala helps keep them focused and gives them a specific way to keep track of time during their meditation.

2. Breathing Techniques

As we mentioned in the previous section on meditation, focusing on your breath can be an excellent way to calm your mind and to deal with both chronic stress and stressful situations as they arise on a day-to-day basis. When our bodies enter the fight or flight response stage, our breathing becomes shallow and rapid. This allows more air to quickly enter our body and gives us the oxygen we will require to run away or stay and fight. If we can learn how to control our breath, we can help stop or slow down the fight or flight reaction in situations where it isn't necessary and learn to deal with stress before it can have a negative effect on us.

Breathing also helps to expel toxins out of our bodies. It is estimated that each time we exhale, we expel approximately 3,500 different compounds. Breathing is a cleansing process that helps to clean our lungs and remove waste from our bodies.

Here are a few breathing techniques that you may find useful when dealing with stressful situations.

- **4-7-8 Technique**

  The 4-7-8 breathing technique has been proven to help during anxiety-causing situations and has even been said to help stop a panic attack in under a minute. To practice this method, follow these steps:

  - Let out a big exhale and remove all of the air from your lungs.
  - Breathe in, counting to 4
  - Hold your breath for the count of 7

- Release your breath very slowly to the count of 8
- Continue this for at least a minute

This technique requires a lot of focus which means that there is very little opportunity for you to focus on anything other than your breath. The rhythmic breathing that this exercise provides can be very calming and soothing and can be used at any time during the day when you feel the effects of stress are getting the better of you.

- **Equal Breathing Technique**

  Similar to the 4-7-8 technique, the equal breathing method helps to level out our breath, especially if stress or anxiety has caused us to have rapid or shallow breathing. Choose a length of time, say, for example, four seconds, and breathe in for that length of time and then immediately breathe out for that same length of time. Breathing in while counting and breathing out while counting will work to slow your breath and invoke a feeling of calm as well.

- **The Wim Hof Method**

  Wim Hof is a Dutch extreme athlete, also known as "The Iceman." He practices a combination of breathing techniques combined with cold therapy to help deal with stress, improve energy levels, enhance sleep, improve focus and willpower, and boost your immune system.

  Wim Hof claims that by learning to master your breath, you will be able to master extreme temperatures. By being able to endure things like cold showers or ice baths. These therapies are said to help speed up your metabolism and burn fat faster, reduce inflammation and pain in the body, improve your immune response, and decrease the symptoms of autoimmune diseases.

  To practice this method:

- Take 30 to 40 deep breaths, inhaling deeply and filling the abdomen, and then exhaling completely.

- When you have completed these breaths, inhale deeply and hold your breath until you have the urge that you need to breathe again.

- When you breathe in, take a deep breath that fills the entire abdomen, chest, and stomach. Hold this breath for approximately 15 seconds and then release it.

- Continue again from the beginning for as many rounds as you would like.

When you have practiced this breathing technique and are comfortable with it, it is time to introduce cold therapy. While under a cold running shower or in a cold bath, continue to perform this steady, rhythmic breathing method. This is supposed to bring about calm, relaxation, and focus to help you deal with the extreme cold temperatures.

3. Yoga

Yoga is an ancient practice that uses different movements and positions, combined with focused breathing techniques to help bring about a sense of calm and relaxation. Yoga is very good at alleviating the effects of stress from our everyday life and has a whole range of other positive benefits.

Yoga can:

- Improve flexibility
- Relieve joint and muscle pain
- Improve balance
- Build muscle
- Reduce inflammation
- Reduce anxiety and boost mood
- Improve digestive health

- Improve cardiovascular health

There are many new yoga studios opening up all over the country with licensed instructors that can assist you. Still, if you prefer, you can also follow along to a YouTube video or yoga app in the comfort of your own home.

4. Tai Chi

Tai Chi is a practice that is very similar to yoga. It combines a very gentle and slow movement with stretching and breathing exercises to promote relaxation, focus, and a feeling of calm. It was originally developed as a form of martial arts in China, but it is now more popularly known as "meditation in motion."

5. Self-Care Time!

One of the very best and easiest ways to combat stress is to find some time, every day for you! Schedule some time to do something that you find relaxing, and make sure that you incorporate it into your day. Take time to read, do a hobby, go for a walk, garden, make a craft or have a relaxing bath. Spending time doing the things you love will clear your mind, improve your mood and relieve any of the effects that chronic stress may be having on your wellbeing.

As you can see, stress is a major factor in both the health of our body and our minds, and learning to deal with it before it takes over is the key to staying vibrant and healthy.

Another key to keeping our immune systems functioning well is taking advantage of some of the many therapies that are available and offered by trained professionals. Let's dive into some of the immune-boosting therapies that can improve our wellness and enhance our immunity.

Chapter Eight
Immune Boosting Therapies

There are so many different things that we can do on our own that can help to improve our health and enhance the functioning of our immune system. We can eat healthy food, take vitamins and supplements, exercise regularly, and manage the stress in our lives. But did you know that there are many different professionals out there who are specifically trained to help us feel better and can implement therapies that can help us fight disease and experience increased immunity?

Most of these therapies can be found in your local communities and can have a profound and lasting impact on your health. Here are just a few of the therapies that could benefit you and your wellbeing.

Where to turn for help with your immune system

- **Naturopath** - A naturopath is a fully trained healthcare professional who specializes in natural therapies and remedies to boost your health and support your immune system. Naturopathy focuses on a completely holistic approach to treating symptoms, cure disease, and boost immunity to prevent future illnesses. Its primary focus is on diet, exercise, supplements, and a combination of other natural therapies to treat the entire body and encourage overall healing.

- **Acupuncture** - Acupuncture is a part of traditional Chinese medicine, and it uses small, metal needles which are placed at key points into the skin. In Chinese medicine, it is believed that we have an energy system called the chi that runs through our body. By inserting acupuncture needles at specific points along this energy system, we can realign our energy and bring about balance to our wellbeing. Acupuncture has been said to relieve pain and inflammation, reduce stress, and improve immune function. It is also relatively risk-free when done by a registered practitioner, so it is an excellent therapy choice for those who cannot find relief with other treatment methods.

- **Massage** - Massage therapy is one of the most widely used alternative therapies. While most people who utilize this method do so for the relaxation and pain-relieving properties it provides, massage also offers many other benefits to the immune system.

  When our muscles and tissues are manually stimulated and massaged, knotted, and tensed areas are relaxed. This improves blood flow and the flow of lymphatic fluid, allowing nutrients to move through the body better and allow toxins to be removed more efficiently. Also, studies have shown a direct link between massage and the number of lymphocytes that our body produces, meaning that after receiving a massage, our bodies are better able to fight off infection.

  The benefits of regular massage include improved pain management, reduced inflammation, improved circulation, better sleep, less stress, better stress management, improved mood, less frequent anxiety, and an overall improved sense of wellbeing.

- **Cupping** - Cupping is a therapy used in Chinese medicine that involves using a heated glass cup that is placed on the skin. The heat creates a vacuum which sucks the skin up into the cup. This method helps to improve immune function by improving circulation and lymphatic fluid flow. Also, because cupping causes a slight skin irritation, it causes a reaction in the body's immune system by causing minor inflammation. This triggers the immune system to go to work producing neutrophils and lymphocytes in the event that the body needs to fend off an attack. This helps to strengthen the overall immune response. People with chronic pain or autoimmune diseases have experienced great results when using the cupping method.

- **Reiki** - Reiki is a Japanese healing technique that combines guided meditation with energy healing to induce relaxation and eliminate stress. It is completely natural and non-invasive and, similar to acupuncture, works to balance a client's energy centers and energy channels to promote self-healing.

  During a Reiki session, a client will lie on a massage table, fully clothed, and will proceed to close their eyes and focus on the gentle flow of their breath. The practitioner will then use calming, guided meditations and a series of light-touch hand positions to bring the client into a state of deep relaxation. The mind begins to slow, and the brainwave pattern will begin to change into the alpha, delta, or theta stages as the session progresses. These stages are when the mind is at its most relaxed and when the body begins to heal and regenerate itself. There are many different activities that will produce the same effects and are conducive to stress reduction, such as meditation, tai chi, and yoga, but Reiki is the only one that takes little to no effort from the client. All that is required is a willingness to attempt to relax and slow your breathing. In fact, it is not uncommon for a client to become so serene that they fall asleep.

- **Chiropractic Care** - When people think of Chiropractors, they often think of doctors cracking their backs and realigning their spines. While this is true, to an extent, chiropractic care offers so many more benefits.

When performed by a licensed professional, a chiropractic adjustment can help treat the musculoskeletal system's disorders, which can help with issues of the nervous system, the reproductive system, the digestive system, and the cardiovascular system. If we are out of alignment, there can be repercussions on so many other parts of the body. Suppose the central nervous system is being negatively affected by our musculoskeletal system. In that case, our immune system will fail to function properly, and the messages that our body sends from one part to another, especially when trying to fight off an illness or disease, won't be received properly.

Regular chiropractic care can reduce pain and allow all of your body's intricate systems to work properly and harmoniously with one another.

- **Colonics** - Colonics is a therapy that many naturopaths and other healthcare professionals recommend. Also known as colon therapy or colonic irrigation, colonics use a solution of water or other fluids which flush out the colon, removing any build-up of waste and any toxins that may be present there.

  Colonics are said to help regulate your bowels, improve your digestive health, improve your body's ability to digest its food, absorb vitamins and minerals, increase energy, and improve your body's ability to lose weight. All of these benefits positively impact your body's microbiome and your immune system's overall health.

- **Aromatherapy** - The science behind aromatherapy is based on the fact that different scents and essential oils have different effects on our bodies. Aromatherapy can be implemented by inhaling certain oils, applying them topically to the skin, or using them as an infusion to a bath.

Aromatherapy has many different benefits. Depending on the specific essential oil you use, you can experience improved sleep, increased energy, reduced pain, improved mood, less frequent headaches, improved nausea, and improved digestive issues. Some essential oils also have antimicrobial, antiviral, antifungal, antibacterial, and antioxidant properties, all of which have a direct, positive effect on the immune system and its ability to function properly and fight disease.

- **Himalayan salt therapy** - Himalayan sea salt is said to contain many different healing properties and health benefits. Just as many people who spend a lot of time by the ocean notice the salt air's benefits, you can get the same benefits by using Himalayan salt therapy.

  Salt rooms are becoming more and more popular and offer participants the chance to sit in a room that is completely filled with Himalayan sea salt. Inches of salt line the floors, and there are slabs of salt crystals throughout the room. Relaxing or meditating in these rooms is extremely beneficial for reducing stress, but the salt's actual effects on the body are profound. Inhaling the salty air is said to cleanse and disinfect the nasal passages, sinuses, throat, and lungs. It can help with chronic lung conditions, allergies, sore throats, asthma, sinus infections, colds, and other viruses. Salt is a natural disinfectant and can help to boost your immunity and provide added support and protection to your immune system.

  If you do not have access to an actual salt room, Himalayan salt lamps and inhalers can be purchased for use at home from most local health food stores.

As you can see, the list of alternative therapies that can boost your health and improve your immune function is quite substantial. When starting your quest for better immunity, it's easy to get overwhelmed, especially when you are trying to learn everything and take on all of the responsibility yourself. There are numerous different professionals and services available that you can take advantage of that will help to improve your health and wellbeing. You can try out a few and stick to the ones that you feel have the most benefit, or you can implement all of them into one comprehensive immune-boosting regimen. The choice is up to you!

Next up, we will explore what happens when our immune system malfunctions and begins to attack our bodies. Autoimmune diseases and food allergies are on the rise in today's society, and next, we will find out why and what we can do to prevent and treat these terrible illnesses.

Sources

- https://www.britannica.com/science/fight-or-flight-response
- https://adrenalfatigue.org/how-stress-makes-it-easier-to-get-and-stay-sick/#:~:text=Here%20is%20how%20chronic%20stress%20directly%20affects%20the,system%20that%20battles%20with%20diseases%20such%20as%20cancer.
- https://www.mayoclinic.org/tests-procedures/acupuncture/about/pac-20392763
- https://www.endocrineweb.com/conditions/adrenal-disorders/adrenal-fatigue
- https://www.healthline.com/health/breathing-exercises-for-anxiety#long-exhal

Chapter Nine
The Rise of Autoimmune Diseases and Food Allergies

The incidence of autoimmune diseases and food allergies is on the rise, and what used to be extremely rare is now a common occurrence among many individuals.

Many studies have found that women are more susceptible to autoimmune diseases than men are, and certain ethnic groups are more likely to get certain autoimmune diseases than others. Some autoimmune diseases seem to be linked to genetics, while others seem to be linked to environmental conditions.

Food allergies, which used to be almost unheard of, are now so prevalent that school systems have had to create new rules about which foods are allowed in the classrooms.

With autoimmune diseases and allergies, the body's immune system essentially malfunctions, causing symptoms and allergic reactions that shouldn't happen with properly functioning immunity. The outcomes can be extremely painful and, in some cases, fatal.

First off, let's take a look at autoimmune diseases.

What is an autoimmune disease?

Our immune systems work to keep our bodies healthy by attacking invading cells such as viruses or bacteria that could potentially make us sick. In the case of an autoimmune disease, our bodies malfunction, and for some reason, our immune systems misfire and begin attacking healthy cells. Some autoimmune diseases attack only a specific organ, while some affect cells all over the entire body. Due to these diseases' nature, they can be very difficult to diagnose and do not have a cure in many cases. Patients with these diseases usually take medications and undergo certain treatments to help manage the symptoms, which often progress, getting worse over time.

What causes an autoimmune disease?

Scientists are unsure what causes an autoimmune disease to occur. Some diseases such as multiple sclerosis and lupus seem to be connected to a genetic dysfunction and often are passed down through heredity. Others may have a link to environmental factors.

Some studies have shown that pollution and exposure to certain chemicals and toxins may have a negative effect on the immune system, causing an autoimmune disease to develop, and others have shown that a poor diet containing high-fat foods or those filled with preservatives could be the culprit. Another theory, called "The Hygiene Theory," proposes that because children are vaccinated against so many illnesses nowadays, they aren't exposed to all of the germs and bacteria that are necessary for the proper development of their immune system. This causes weaker overall immunity and causes their immune system to overreact in the future and begin attacking itself.

The 6 most common autoimmune disorders

There are approximately 80 different types of autoimmune diseases that are known today. Many of them have very similar signs and symptoms, which can often make diagnosing them extremely difficult. Below we will take a look at some of the most common.

1. Rheumatoid arthritis

Also known as RA, this disease primarily affects the joints of the wrist and hands. It can be extremely debilitating and painful, causing severe swelling and inflammation and making daily tasks nearly impossible. The immune system begins to attack the joints' tissue and muscles, which causes pain and sometimes disfigurement.

In recent years, many new medical advancements have made a living with rheumatoid arthritis much more manageable, slowing its progression and decreasing the discomfort caused by this disease. RA is more common in women and, in most cases, is seen in people over the age of 50.

2. Lupus

In many cases, lupus can be very difficult to diagnose because it affects many different parts of the body. Each person who is affected may experience a different set of symptoms. One of the most telling signs of this disease is a butterfly-shaped rash that spreads across the face. This autoimmune disease causes inflammation that can affect the skin, joints, kidneys, heart, lungs, and brain.

Because this disease is systemic and affects the entire body, it can be very dangerous and often fatal. Lupus is most common in women between the ages of 15 and 45 who are of African American, Asian and Hispanic descent. It also appears to be hereditary, and those with an incidence of this disease in their family history are at a greater risk of developing it themselves.

3. Psoriasis

This autoimmune disorder affects the skin by causing skin cells to grow much more rapidly than they should. This rapid growth causes the skin cells to build up in scaly, white, or silver patches called plaque. It can occur anywhere on the body and can be itchy or painful. Some cases may only affect a very small area of skin, while more severe cases can affect the entire body. Psoriasis is not contagious, and while there is no cure, its symptoms can be treated with topical solutions, oral medications, or injections.

4. Type 1 diabetes

There are approximately 1.3 million people in the United States living with Type 1 diabetes. This disease occurs when the beta cells in the pancreas stop producing insulin. While the exact cause is unknown, the immune system turns on the body and begins to destroy the cells responsible for producing insulin. Insulin is a hormone that is necessary for the proper metabolism of sugar in the bloodstream. When our bodies do not produce enough of this hormone, there is no way for the sugar that we eat to exit the bloodstream and enter the cells where it is supposed to be used for energy. Telltale signs of Type 1 diabetes include high blood glucose levels, frequent urination, excessive thirst, and weight loss.

Currently, the only way to manage Type 1 diabetes is through multiple insulin injections, frequent blood glucose tests throughout the day, and mindful eating and carbohydrate counting to ensure the proper amount of sugar intake.

5. Hashimoto's disease

Hashimoto's disease is an autoimmune disorder that affects the thyroid gland. This gland produces hormones that are vital for the proper functioning of numerous different systems throughout the body. With Hashimoto's disease, the thyroid becomes inflamed, which leads to an imbalance of hormone production and causes many different symptoms such as tiredness, sensitivity to cold temperatures, unusual weight gain, pale skin, weakness, joint pain, hoarse voice, and swelling of the thyroid gland. This disease is usually easily manageable with prescription thyroid medications.

6. Multiple Sclerosis

Also known as MS, Multiple Sclerosis is an autoimmune disease that occurs when the body's immune system starts attacking the central nervous system. The myelin that surrounds our nerve cells begins to deteriorate, which can cause symptoms such as vision problems, numbness and tingling, muscle spasm and muscle weakness, difficulty moving, and extreme fatigue. MS is most common in women and is usually diagnosed between the ages of 20 - 40.

Some other common autoimmune diseases include:

- Crohn's Disease
- Graves Disease
- Addison's Disease
- Endometriosis
- Fibromyalgia
- Guilaine-Barré Syndrome
- Restless Leg Syndrome
- Narcolepsy

The medical and scientific communities have spent a great deal of time researching the causes of autoimmune disorders in recent years. They are making great advancements in understanding their origins and causes. Treatment options are now more widely available, and although there are no cures yet, new discoveries in areas such as stem cell treatment are paving the road for a brighter future, free from autoimmune disorders.

Tips to prevent autoimmune diseases

While there is no proven method to guarantee that you or your family members will never get an autoimmune disease, there are some things that you can do to help minimize your risk and boost up your immune system.

Take care of your gut - We have already learned how important our gut health is in terms of having strong immunity. By boosting your gut health, you can ensure that your body is digesting the food you eat properly and absorbing all of the minerals you eat. This helps to protect both your microbiome and your entire immune system, reducing the chances that you will be affected by an autoimmune disease.

Minimize your exposure to toxic chemicals - We are exposed to toxic chemicals every day of our lives. From toxins in the air that we breathe, the food that we eat, and the products that we use, it's almost impossible to completely eliminate the chemicals that we are exposed to and improve our immune system's health and protect ourselves against autoimmune diseases we should try. Purchase organic foods that are antibiotic and pesticide-free and use natural cleaning products and personal care products in your home. Many of these products can be made at home using completely natural ingredients or can be purchased at your local health food store.

Eat a healthy diet - The food we eat is the fuel that our bodies use to keep us healthy and keep our bodies functioning properly. Make sure that your diet contains a wide variety of different whole foods that are packed with nutrients.

Maintain a healthy weight - Eating a healthy diet is an important step in this process, and so is getting regular exercise. Both of these combined will help to keep your weight in check and reduce an added strain on your immune system.

Support your immune system with supplements - We have already looked at a whole list of vitamins, minerals, and supplements that can help to protect your immune system. Talk to your healthcare provider about which supplements are best for you and which can best help to keep your immune system strong and healthy.

Fight off any infections early on - Exposure to certain viruses and bacteria is another potential cause of autoimmune diseases. If you find yourself feeling under the weather, seek your healthcare provider's assistance and start treatment right away. Also, in the event that you do develop an autoimmune disease one day, early diagnosis and treatment is one of the best ways to manage your symptoms and slow the disease's progression.

Stop your bad habits - We have all heard it a million times before; smoking, drinking, and drugs are all bad for us. They can weaken our immune systems and make us much more susceptible to a whole host of other diseases, including autoimmune disease.

Now let's take a peek at how the immune system plays an important role in the development of food allergies.

What is a food allergy?

Like an autoimmune disease, a food allergy occurs when the body mistakenly identifies a food as a harmful invader. It is usually one of the proteins in a food that causes the body to react, sending out different symptoms, some of which are quite mild and some which can be extremely dangerous and life-threatening.

What are the different types of food allergies?

There are two main types of food allergies, IgE and IgG. Both of these have to do with the immune system's response to food, but one has much more serious consequences than the other.

IgE Food Allergy - Immunoglobulin E is an antibody that the body's immune system produces when it feels that the body may be under threat from a foreign body or substance. When you eat a specific food, the body quickly releases this antibody which causes a very severe and immediate allergic reaction called anaphylaxis. Even with minimal exposure to the allergy-causing food, the symptoms can be quite severe and require medical intervention. The use of an Epi-pen is often required.

Symptoms of this type of allergic reaction include:

- Hives
- Swelling of the lips, eyes, face, and hands
- Itching
- Difficulty breathing

- Difficulty swallowing
- Nausea
- Vomiting
- Diarrhea
- Dizziness
- Skin or lips turning blue.
- Weak pulse

Usually, an IgE allergy is discovered too late after exposure to a specific food source. However, blood tests can be done to diagnose or confirm these types of allergies. Some of the most common food sources that cause these allergies are tree nuts, legumes, seafood, wheat, eggs, and milk.

IgG Food Allergy - Immunoglobulin G is responsible for IgG food allergies, which is more accurately referred to as food intolerances or sensitivities. This response occurs when our body's immune system produces a much subtler and less severe reaction, often in the form of increased inflammation, when we eat a specific food.

When we suffer from symptoms of an allergic reaction to something we ate or came into contact with but are unsure of the cause, IgG food intolerances may be the culprit. Symptoms do not usually occur immediately and may take up to a few days to appear.

Some of the common symptoms of an IgG food allergy include:

- Headaches
- Bloating
- Gas
- Diarrhea
- Acid reflux
- Anxiety
- Depression
- Fatigue
- Memory or concentration issues

Your healthcare provider can offer a simple blood test that can check for some of the most common IgG food allergies (such as dairy, gluten, eggs, and certain vegetables and fruits), and by minimizing or completely eliminating exposure to these foods, you should be able to avoid any symptoms of the allergy.

Autoimmune diseases and food allergies give us a bit of insight into how important it is to take care of our immune system and ensure that it is working properly to protect us from outside invaders instead of turning on our own bodies instead. It should go without saying that if we take better care of our bodies, our bodies will take better care of us. While not all allergies and autoimmune diseases are preventable, by nurturing and nourishing our bodies properly, we will be able to experience a lower incidence of disease and less severe symptoms of illness throughout our lifetimes.

Next, we will take a look at one specific illness that shook the world and, in a very short amount of time, has changed the way that we live - the Coronavirus.

Sources

- https://www.healthline.com/health/autoimmune-disorders
- https://www.niehs.nih.gov/health/topics/conditions/autoimmune/index.cfm
- https://foodallergycanada.ca/food-allergy-basics/food-allergies-101/what-are-food-allergies/
- https://foodallergycanada.ca/food-allergy-basics/preventing-and-treating-allergic-reactions/reaction-signs-and-symptoms/?gclid=Cj0KCQiA4L2BBhCvARIsAO0SBdbZwUx5bPWKcQ0RJmT8jwnYz9p1WHx81pZzVCkFuDQEB4XHX64x-MaAsOFEALwwcB

Chapter Ten
Don't Be Afraid of The Big, Bad Coronavirus

In early 2020, rumors of a terrible virus that started in Wuhan, China, began spreading across the globe, and not long after, the actual virus began spreading as well. The media was consumed with horror stories of a deadly virus that was sweeping the globe and could wipe us all out in one single, horrifying blow.

Now that things have finally calmed down, studies have been conducted, and we are now able to look at the entire situation objectively. Is the Coronavirus as scary as we have been lead to believe? The answer is: Yes and no.

As with any virus, the Coronavirus can be extremely deadly, especially for those people who already have a compromised immune system. Senior citizens, people who have any type of autoimmune disease, those who are overweight or consume an unhealthy diet or have heart disease, respiratory issues, or any kind of cancer are at much greater risk of contracting a severe and even fatal case of this disease. Becoming sick with any virus or bacteria could be an extremely dangerous situation for someone whose immune system has already been compromised by another illness. Proof of this can be seen every year during cold and flu season. Thousands of people are hospitalized, and thousands die from the flu every year.

Many reports say that COVID-19 (the disease caused by the current Coronavirus) is much deadlier than the seasonal flu, with a fatality of 2%. However, this number is hard to calculate because all too often, people who have mild cases of COVID-19 don't seek medical treatment. The death rate statistic will appear much higher because it only considers the most severe cases that require medical assistance. Many people, especially those under 40 years old, have gotten the virus and recovered from it without needing any medical attention. Many people in this same age demographic have contracted the virus but showed no symptoms because their immune system was able to fight it off before it made them sick. Most people who become ill will be able to successfully fight off the virus at home and take natural or over-the-counter remedies to treat their symptoms. Due to these facts, the actual numbers being reported are grossly inaccurate.

What is the Coronavirus?

Did you know that there are over 100 different types of coronaviruses that have been identified? Many of the coronaviruses that we are aware of only infect animals, while others can be transmitted from animals to humans.

The coronaviruses are all transmitted the same way, through droplets of bodily fluids that are expelled from an infected person by coughing or sneezing. These droplets travel through the air and can either be inhaled or contaminate a surface where they can be transferred via touch and ingested.

A person may be infected for between two and fourteen days before they begin showing symptoms which means that the virus can be transmitted to other people who have no idea that they have been exposed to this virus.

The first cases of coronaviruses were discovered in the 1960s and are classified into four different groups: alpha, beta, gamma, and delta. The alpha and beta types primarily affect mammals, while the gamma and delta strains affect birds. These viruses are made up of a strip of genetic material called RNA that is surrounded by proteins that stick up like tiny spikes. Under a microscope, these little spikes appear to look like a crown. This is where the virus got its name. Corona in Latin translates to crown.

The symptoms that you experience will differ slightly depending on the type of Coronavirus that you have been exposed to. Some affect the nasal passages only, causing mild symptoms, while others will attack the lower parts of the lungs, making them more difficult to treat and causing much more severe and life-threatening symptoms.

Let's take a look at some of the most common coronaviruses.

MERS - Which stands for Middle East Respiratory Syndrome, is a type of Coronavirus that is transmitted from camels to humans. It was first discovered in 2012 in Saudi Arabia. MERS attacks the respiratory system, causing shortness of breath, leading to severe pneumonia and possibly kidney failure. Four out of every ten reported cases of this virus have died.

SARS - Which stands for Severe Acute Respiratory Syndrome, was first reported in Asia in early 2003. This virus quickly spread worldwide, and in 2003, there was an outbreak that affected a reported 8,098 people across the globe. During this outbreak, 774 people lost their lives.

SARS infection usually begins with a high fever leading to a cough and often nausea and diarrhea. Most severe cases of SARS lead to pneumonia.

H1N1 - In 2009, the H1N1 virus began spreading across the world, and between April 2009 to April 2010, there were an estimated 60 million cases, 270,000 hospitalizations, and 12,469 deaths in the United States alone from this virus.

This particular virus is spread from pigs to humans and is also known as the swine flu. What made this virus unique is that the majority of the people who were severely affected were under the age of 65. Due to other very similar viruses that were present in the past, much of the older population had already developed immunity from past exposure. It, therefore, was able to fight off this new strain much easier.

Avian Flu - The avian flu often only infects aquatic birds, but this virus can be spread to domestic birds like chickens. When this happens, it can then be passed on to humans, causing outbreaks of illness. Over the years, there have been many outbreaks around this type of Coronavirus. In 2004 we saw the largest outbreak of this virus that spread across many Asian countries.

What can I do to prevent the Coronavirus?

As with any viral infection, one of the best ways to remain healthy is to prevent catching the virus in the first place. By maintaining good personal hygiene and keeping your immune system strong and healthy, you can protect yourself from becoming infected.

Here are some of the top tips for avoiding the Coronavirus:

- **Wash your hands** - I know you have heard this one before but washing your hands is one of the best ways to keep from getting any type of virus. Viruses can live for extended periods of time on hard surfaces and can easily be transferred to your hands. These viruses can easily enter your system if you touch your eyes or mouth or the food you eat.

- **Get lots of rest** - We have already talked about the importance of sleep but getting lots of rest, especially during cold and flu season or during a pandemic, can mean the difference between getting sick and staying healthy.

- **Distance yourself from those who are sick** - Keeping a safe distance from others, especially those who are sick, will help to keep you from getting sick as well. The droplets of body fluid, which carry the Coronavirus, can travel up to six feet, so being closer than this distance to someone who has contracted the virus would obviously increase your risk of contracting the virus yourself. Also, studies have shown that being in contact with an infected person for longer than fifteen minutes will significantly increase your risk factor as well.

- **Eat a healthy, whole-food diet** - As we have discussed before, one of the best ways to keep your immune system strong and ready to fight off any intruding viral attacks is to eat a healthy, balanced diet. A bright and colorful diet that is filled with lots of plant-based food is low in saturated fats, refined sugars, and processed foods will provide your body with tons of nutrients, vitamins, minerals, and fiber. They will support your immune system, keeping it functioning properly.

- **Boost your immunity with supplements** - Sometimes, it is impossible to get all of the vitamins and minerals that your body requires from the foods you eat. Taking a daily dose of vitamins, minerals and supplements is an excellent way to stay healthy and strong.

  Some supplements have been proven to have a higher level of success in boosting your immune system and reduce your risk of contracting the Coronavirus. Some of these supplements that should be added to your anti-Coronavirus regiment should include:

  - **Vitamin D3** - This vitamin has some excellent immune-supporting properties and can help decrease inflammation while assisting white blood cells in attacking invaders. Studies have shown that most people do not get enough vitamin D3. So, in the age of COVID 19, taking a daily dose of a highly potent form of vitamin D3 will do you a world of good.

- **Zinc** - Zinc helps to support your immune system and is essential for immune cells to develop and grow properly. Studies have shown that taking this supplement can help prevent illness, and if you are already sick, taking zinc can help decrease the length and severity of the illness.

- **Vitamin C** - This vitamin is probably the first to come to mind when you think of enhancing immunity and staying healthy. Vitamin C helps to reduce oxidation in the cells of the body, keeping them from deteriorating or dying off early. This vitamin also protects you from getting sick and will equip your immune system to fight off an illness if you become sick.

- **Elderberry** - This supplement is being investigated for its ability to reduce the symptoms and severity of upper respiratory tract infections. It also has strong antiviral and antibiotic properties that help the immune system fend off pending attacks.

- **Neem** - Is one of the most popular herbs in the world of Ayurveda. It has an array of medicinal properties that help keeping you away from common infections. It has over 130 biologically active compounds that have been shown to actively fight of viruses and bacterial diseases. While there are no clinical studies linking Neem with COVID 19 it has been proven to build up a person's natural immunity to contracting the disease. It has also been shown to aide in a speedier recovery from COVID 19 as well. It is particularly effective when it is taken in combination with Turmeric which is a herb that has been proven to reduce inflammation which is one of the major symptoms of COVID 19 and all coronaviruses that cause acute inflammation of the lungs.

- **Hydroxychloroquine** – Despite all the controversy that surrounded the use of this drug as a prophylactic, treatment or even cure for COVID 19, research later showed that it is indeed a very effective and safe medical weapon to fight this deadly virus.

  According to Wikipedia: Hydroxychloroquine was approved for medical use in the United States in 1955. It is on the WHO's list of essential medicines. In 2017, it was the 128th most commonly prescribed medication in the United States, with more than five million prescriptions.

  Clinical studies showed that treatment with hydroxychloroquine cut the death rate significantly in sick patients hospitalized with COVID-19 – and without heart-related side-effects, according to a new study published by the Henry Ford Health System.

  In a large-scale retrospective analysis of 2,541 patients hospitalized between March 10 and May 2, 2020 across the system's six hospitals, the study found 13% of those treated with hydroxychloroquine alone died compared to 26.4% not treated with hydroxychloroquine. None of the patients had documented serious heart abnormalities; however, patients were monitored for a heart condition routinely pointed to as a reason to avoid the drug as a treatment for COVID-19.

  The study was published in the International Journal of Infectious Diseases, the peer-reviewed, open-access online publication of the International Society of Infectious Diseases (ISID.org).

- **Ivermectin** – Similar controversy has surrounded the use of this drug as an effective treatment for those who have contracted COVID 19. Ivermectin has been used for more than 30 years for the treatment of several diseases. More than one million doses of the drug are administered daily, particularly in low- and middle-income countries. Due to the low prevalence of adverse events with the use of this drug, ivermectin is considered to have a good safety profile and its potential benefit in other diseases is currently under investigation.

  An in vitro study of ivermectin in SARS-CoV-2 in Australia showed a significant reduction of viral load in infected cells. Subsequently, a descriptive study of 704 critical patients with COVID-19 showed a reduction in mortality, hospitalization, and intensive care unit length-of-stay in those patients who received the drug. Unfortunately, this study was withdrawn by its authors, leaving more questions than answers.

  Some countries in Latin America have authorized its use for the management of patients with COVID-19 even in the absence of solid evidence, and several other countries are conducting clinical trials to evaluate its efficacy for the treatment of moderate and severe disease.

What are the symptoms of the Coronavirus?

The Coronavirus can present with any combination of the following list of symptoms:

- Fever

- Fatigue
- Dry cough
- Loss of appetite
- Body Aches
- Shortness of breath
- Excess mucus
- Sore throat
- Chills
- Headache
- Loss of Taste
- Loss of Smell
- Congestion
- Runny nose
- Nausea
- Vomiting
- Diarrhea
- Pink eye
- Skin rash

Many people who get Coronavirus will get only a few symptoms if any, while others may exhibit many. Some of these symptoms can lead to more serious liver failure complications, kidney damage, heart failure, seizures, and blood clots.

How can I treat COVID-19 if I become sick?

If you find yourself experiencing any of the symptoms of the Coronavirus, you can try these helpful tips to speed up your recovery time and get feeling back to normal as quickly as possible:

- **Drink lots of fluids** - Staying hydrated is important, especially when you are sick. While you may not feel like drinking much, forcing yourself to meet the daily recommended fluid intake of eight cups a day will help you stay healthy and strong and keep you from experiencing dehydration symptoms on top of the symptoms of COVID-19 as well.

- **Get lots of rest** - Our body uses the time that we rest to recover. It is then that our immune cells function best and are better able to fight off an infection. Getting as much rest as possible will help us to recover much faster. Many people may get the urge to push themselves and try to get back to their usual routine as quickly as possible, but this will only add undue stress to your body and force your immune system to have to work harder.

- **Take your vitamins** - Make sure that you still keep up on your daily regimen of vitamins and minerals when you are sick. This will ensure that your body still gets the nutrients that it needs, especially if you don't have a strong appetite and aren't eating as much as usual.

- **Use honey and lemon to soothe your cough** - If you are suffering from a sore throat or cough, the combination of honey and lemon (especially in a tea) is excellent for soothing the throat, relieving congestion, and it has antibacterial and antiviral properties to help eliminate the pathogens that are making you sick.

If you are at high risk for developing complications from COVID-19 or at any time you are having difficulty breathing or feel extremely ill, call your local health department 911 or visit your nearest hospital for medical treatment immediately.

As with any illness, the Coronavirus should not be taken lightly, but that being said, it should not be feared any more than any other virus either. Ensuring that you do everything you can to bolster up your immunity will help you stay healthy and stay safe from COVID-19 and any other illness you may encounter.

If you are looking for even more ways to heighten your level of immunity, read on and try out some of these amazing recipes that are chock full of nutrients and health-boosting properties.

Sources

- https://www.webmd.com/lung/covid-19-symptoms#1
- https://www.cdc.gov/coronavirus/mers/index.html
- https://www.cdc.gov/flu/pandemic-resources/2009-h1n1-pandemic.html
- https://www.cdc.gov/flu/avianflu/index.htm
- https://www.canada.ca/en/health-canada/services/healthy-living/your-health/diseases/avian-influenza-bird-flu.html
- https://www.healthline.com/nutrition/immune-boosting-supplements#1.-Vitamin-D
- https://www.india.com/lifestyle/neem-can-help-you-in-fight-against-coronavirus-here-is-how-4035383/
- https://en.wikipedia.org/wiki/Hydroxychloroquine
- https://www.ijidonline.com/article/S1201-9712(20)30534-8/fulltext
- https://www.henryford.com
- https://isid.org/2019-novel-coronavirus/
- https://clinicaltrials.gov/ct2/show/NCT04602507

Chapter Eleven
Immune Boosting Diet Plan

Eating healthy, nutrient-rich foods is one of the most important things that we can do to boost our immunity and increase our gut health. There are so many nutrient-rich foods available to us that can provide us with all of the nutrition that our body needs to function properly and work hard to keep us healthy and disease-free.

In this chapter, we have put together a collection of some of the best immune-boosting recipes that should be to your meal plan.

Bon Appetit!

CHICKEN SOUP

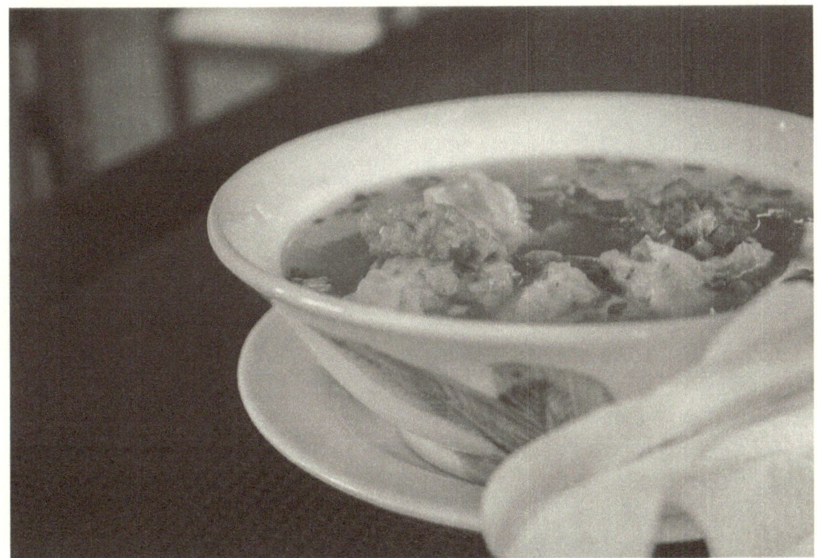

Chicken soup is a staple for cold and flu season, and for good reason! Not only is it warm and soothing when we are feeling under the weather, but it also provides an arsenal of virus-fighting and immune-boosting properties. Studies have shown that chicken soup helps to reduce inflammation, relieve congestion, has antibacterial properties, and provides vitamins, minerals, and protein that can help to amp up your immune system and give your body the energy that it needs to ward off sickness and disease. Whether you are already sick or looking for a soup that will help keep you healthy, this recipe has it all!

Ingredients

6 medium carrots, chopped

6 celery stalks, chopped

5 garlic cloves, minced

1 medium onion, chopped

1.5 lbs. Pre-cooked chicken, chopped into cubes

2 tbsp Italian spices

¼ tsp dried thyme

2 tsp dried rosemary

8 cups chicken bone broth

Water as needed to fill the pot

1 tsp sea salt

1 tsp black pepper

Fresh basil or cilantro for garnishing

Avocado oil for cooking

Directions

1. In a large pot, place the carrots, celery, and avocado oil on medium heat. Cook for 10 minutes to soften.

2. Add the garlic and onions and cook for an additional 5 minutes.

3. Next, add the pre-cooked, chopped chicken, Italian spices, thyme, rosemary, broth, water, salt, and pepper.

4. Let the pot simmer for 20 minutes to take on all the flavor.

5. Top with fresh herbs like basil or cilantro.

6. If you would like to add some spice, you can add in some red pepper flakes. This has the added bonus of helping to relieve congestion.

Enjoy!

ROASTED GARLIC, TOMATO, AND RED PEPPER SOUP

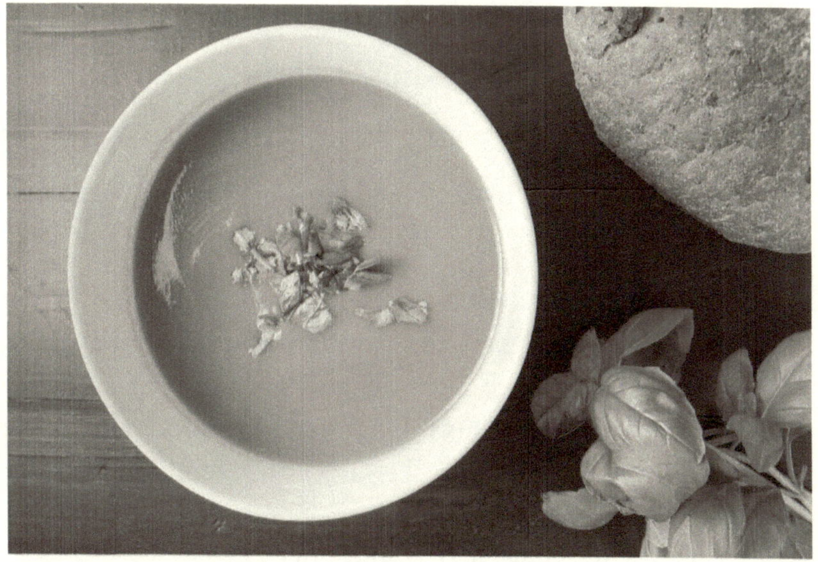

This soup is full of all kinds of immune-boosting goodness! It is jam-packed with vitamin C and lycopene from the tomatoes and red peppers, and the roasted garlic is a natural antibacterial and antifungal agent.

Ingredients

2 lbs. Fresh on-the-vine tomatoes, quartered

1 large red pepper, stem and seeds removed and roughly chopped

1 small yellow onion, roughly chopped

1 small head garlic, halved widthwise

2 tbsp olive oil

½ tsp dried basil

½ tsp thyme

1 tbsp coconut sugar

1 cup full fat coconut milk

1 ½ - 2 cups vegetable broth

A small handful of fresh dill, roughly chopped

¼ tsp red pepper flakes for extra spice (optional)

Salt and pepper to taste

Directions

1. Preheat the oven to 425°F and line a large baking sheet with parchment paper.

2. Spread the quartered tomatoes, red pepper, and onion on the baking sheet and place the halved garlic pieces in the center. Drizzle evenly with olive oil, and sprinkle with basil and thyme. Season generously with salt and pepper and gently toss together. Make sure the garlic is lying cut side down on the baking sheet. Roast for 35 minutes until tomatoes and peppers are lightly charred and cooked down.

3. While the vegetables are roasting, heat the coconut milk and vegetable broth in a pot over medium heat. When the vegetables are done roasting, squeeze the caramelized garlic out of its skin, and transfer to a high-speed blender with the vegetables, hot liquid mixture, and the remaining ingredients.

4. Blend on high speed until completely smooth and creamy. Taste and season with more salt and pepper if necessary. Serve hot with a drizzle of olive oil, a pinch of pepper flakes, and fresh dill.

Enjoy!

ROASTED VEGETABLE CURRY BOWL

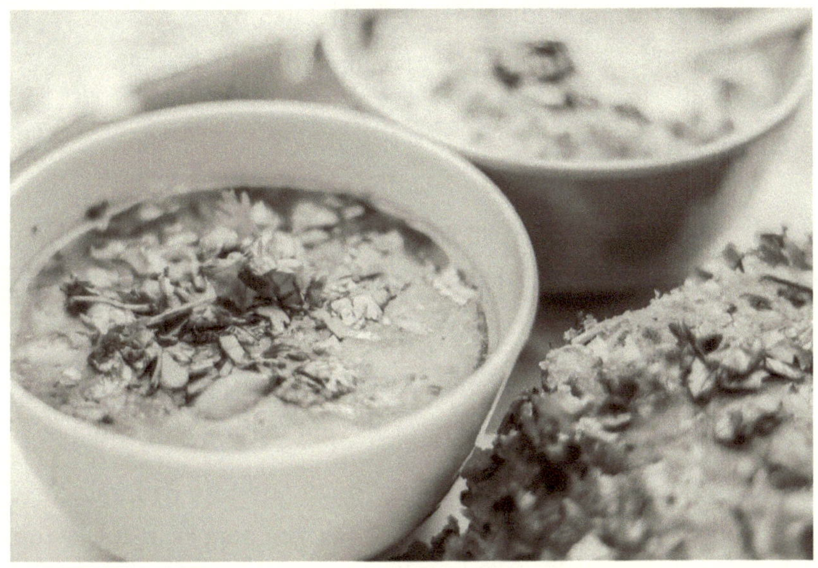

Are you looking to boost up your immunity and rev up the health of your gut's microbiome as well? This delicious curry bowl has everything you need! This high-fiber recipe is full of vegetables and legumes, which will help fuel your microbiome. Plus, as an added bonus, the butternut squash in this dish still has the skin on! It is completely edible when roasted and contains tons of extra fiber, vitamins, and minerals!

Ingredients

Vegetables

½ medium butternut squash

1 large cooking onion

2 large carrots

½ small head cauliflower

2 tbsp mild curry powder

½ tsp coriander seeds, ground

½ cup mung dahl beans

1 tsp mild curry

⅛ tsp coriander seeds, ground

¼ tsp cumin

1 tsp maple syrup

1 cup canned coconut milk

½ tsp fresh ginger, grated

½ tbsp maple syrup

½ tbsp avocado oil

2 cloves garlic, minced

Mung Dahl

1 garlic clove, minced

Toppings

Fresh cilantro

Cultured vegetables

Directions

1. Preheat oven to 400°F. Slice squash in half, scoop out insides, and slice half of the squash into thin slices, leaving the skin on.

2. Cut cauliflower, onions, and carrots into large chunky pieces. This helps them cook evenly with the squash pieces.

3. Place vegetables into a large bowl and toss with oil. Next, sprinkle on spices, a pinch of salt and pepper, maple syrup, and minced garlic. Stir well and pour vegetables onto a lined cookie tray. Place into the oven and cook for 22-30 minutes until the vegetables' edges are a little browned.

4. While vegetables are just in the oven, place mung dal beans into a saucepan with 1 ½ cups water. Bring to a boil and add a pinch of salt and pepper. Cover and turn down to simmer for 15 minutes. Then uncover, stir, and add garlic, fresh ginger, maple syrup, coconut milk from a can, and spices. Stir and keep on simmer, uncovered, stirring often until mixture thickens and dahl is soft.

5. To assemble, place roasted vegetables into bowls, top with dahl coconut mixture, fresh cilantro, and cultured vegetables. Serve hot.

Enjoy!

KIMCHI

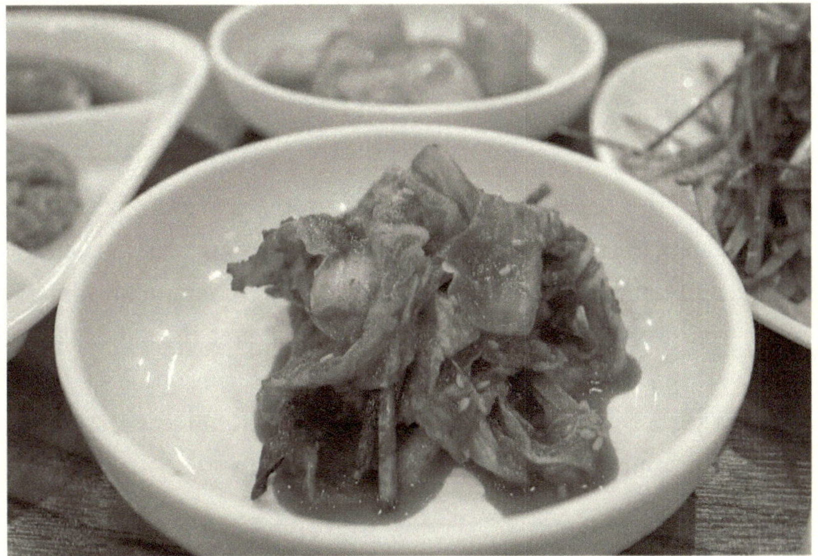

Kimchi is a Korean dish that is made with fermented vegetables. This food is alive with good bacteria and probiotics that will help support your gut's microbiome, plus it tastes delicious and can be used as a side with any meal or as a topper for your salads!

Ingredients

2 pounds napa cabbage, cored and cut into 1-inch pieces (one large cabbage)

¼ cup sea salt

2 cups daikon radish, cut into matchstick strips (optional, or use carrots)

1 bunch scallions, trimmed and cut into 1-inch pieces

1 tablespoon fresh ginger, sliced (2-3 disks, peels ok)

6 cloves garlic, whole

1 shallot, quartered (optional)

2-6 tablespoons Korean-style red pepper flakes

2 tablespoons fish sauce (or you can use vegan fish sauce, miso paste, or soy sauce), more to taste

2 teaspoons sugar (or an alternative like honey, brown rice syrup)

Directions

1. Salt the cabbage. Reserve 1-2 outer leaves of the napa cabbage and refrigerate for later use (wrap in plastic). Cut the remaining cabbage and place it in a large bowl with the salt, and toss. Add enough cool water to cover the cabbage and stir until salt is dissolved. Keep the cabbage submerged with a plate over the bowl and let stand at room temperature for 6-8 hours, giving a stir midway through.

2. Drain the cabbage, saving the brine. Rinse the cabbage quickly, drain, squeeze out any excess water, or blot with paper towels, and place it back in the bowl, adding the daikon radish and scallions.

3. Make the paste. Place the ginger, garlic, shallot, red pepper flakes, fish sauce (or alternatives), and sugar in your food processor. Process until well combined, pulsing until it becomes a thick paste.

4. Scoop the paste over the cabbage, and using tongs or gloved hands, mix and massage the vegetables and the red pepper mixture together really well, until well coated.

5. Pack the cabbage into a large, two-quart jar, leaving 1-2 inches room at the top for juices to release. Add a little of the reserved brine to just cover the vegetables, pressing them down a bit (so they are submerged). Place the whole cabbage leaf over the top, pressing down, which will help keep the kimchi submerged under the brine. You can also use a fermentation weight placed over the whole leaf's top to keep it submerged.

6. Cover loosely with a lid (allowing air to escape and place the jar in a baking dish (or big bowl) to collect any juices that may escape. Leave this somewhere dark and cool for 3 days. A basement or lower cooler cabinet in the pantry or kitchen, away from appliances or heat sources, works best.

7. On the evening of day 3, check for the fermentation action of bubbles. Tap the jar and see if tiny bubbles rise to the top. Check for overflow (which also indicates fermentation). If you see bubbles, it is ready to store in the refrigerator, where it will continue to ferment and develop more flavor slowly. For a softer, tangier kimchi, you can continue to ferment for 3 more days or longer. If no action, give it another day or two. If you don't see bubbles when tapping the jar, it may just need a few more days, especially in cooler climates. Be patient!

8. After you have seen bubbles (usually after 3-5 days), the kimchi is ready, but it won't achieve its full flavor and complexity until about 2 weeks in the fridge, once it has had the chance to ferment slowly. The longer you ferment, the more complex and tangy the taste. If you like a fizzy brine, tighten the lid, burping every week or so. If you don't want to think about it, give the lid one loose twist, leaving room for gasses to escape.

9. This kimchi will keep for months on end in the fridge as long as it is submerged in the brine and will continue to ferment very slowly, getting more and more flavorful.

10. Serve the kimchi as a side dish, on rice, in burritos, on top of salads, or on top of the soup.

Enjoy!

HOMEMADE YOGURT

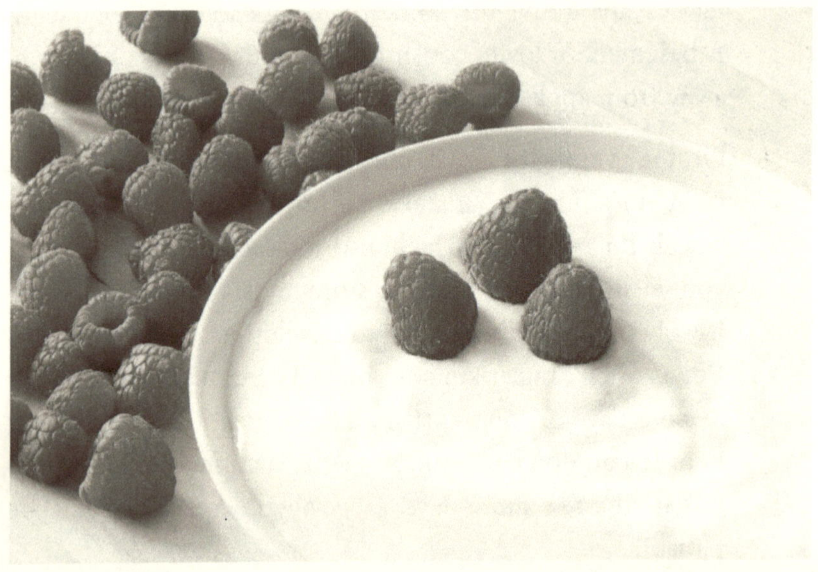

What better way to boost your gut health and power-up your microbiome than with a creamy batch of homemade yogurt! This recipe is overflowing with good bacteria and enzymes that will help with your digestion and provide lots of support to your immune system. It can be eaten on its own or used as a dressing or dip by adding your own blend of spices!

Ingredients

½ gallon raw organic milk

3-4 T unsweetened yogurt from the grocery store with active live cultures (or yogurt from a previous batch)

Cheesecloth

Thermometer

1. Turn oven on to the lowest setting for 10 minutes. Turn off, but leave the light on.

2. Heat milk gently in a pot on the stove. If you want all the benefits of raw milk yogurt, remember to heat the milk only to 110 degrees and no higher. This ensures that milk's own bacteria will stay alive. Or, if unsure, heat to 180F. (please see notes)

3. Add 3-4 tablespoons of yogurt. (The general rule is 2 tablespoons yogurt per quart of milk) Resist the temptation to add more or end up with yogurt that is watery and sour. Cover, wrap in a towel, and place in the oven with the light on or the oven on the lowest setting for a short period of time. The light will act as an incubator.

4. You could also place on a heating pad on the lowest setting. The idea is to keep the yogurt at a steady but low warmth (100F-110F) for a period of 8 hours. If it gets too warm, it will curdle.

5. After 8 hours, strain with a cheesecloth. Store in an airtight container in the fridge. Once cooled, it is ready to eat.

6. If you like sweetened yogurt, mix in honey, vanilla, maple, or agave.

7. I prefer to sweeten yogurt in smaller batches, keeping my main batch plain.

Enjoy!

IMMUNE SHOT

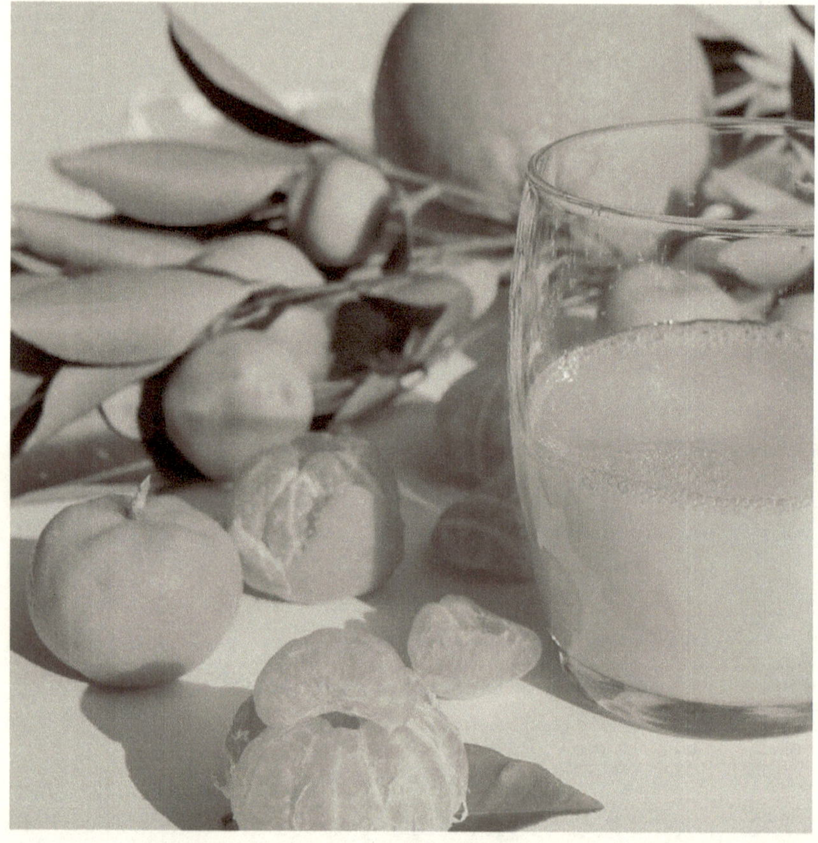

This tiny shot packs a big punch! It contains a concentrated amount of immune-boosting ingredients that will help to keep you from getting sick or can help you fight off an infection if you feel yourself getting sick.

Ingredients

1 tablespoon honey

Juice of 1 lemon

Juice of 1 navel orange

1-2 cloves garlic minced and set aside 10 m

1 teaspoon fresh ginger grated

Dash of cayenne pepper

Dash of real sea salt

Dash cinnamon

1/4 teaspoon turmeric

Grind of black pepper

1 tablespoon organic apple cider vinegar

1 tablespoon hot water

Directions

1. Mince the garlic (ideally put through a garlic press) and set aside for 10 minutes. This gives the enzymes a chance to form and ensures maximum benefits.

2. Whisk together the honey, turmeric, and hot water, until the honey is incorporated and smooth.

3. Stir in remaining ingredients and drink!

APPLE CIDER VINEGAR AND LEMON HAYMAKER'S PUNCH

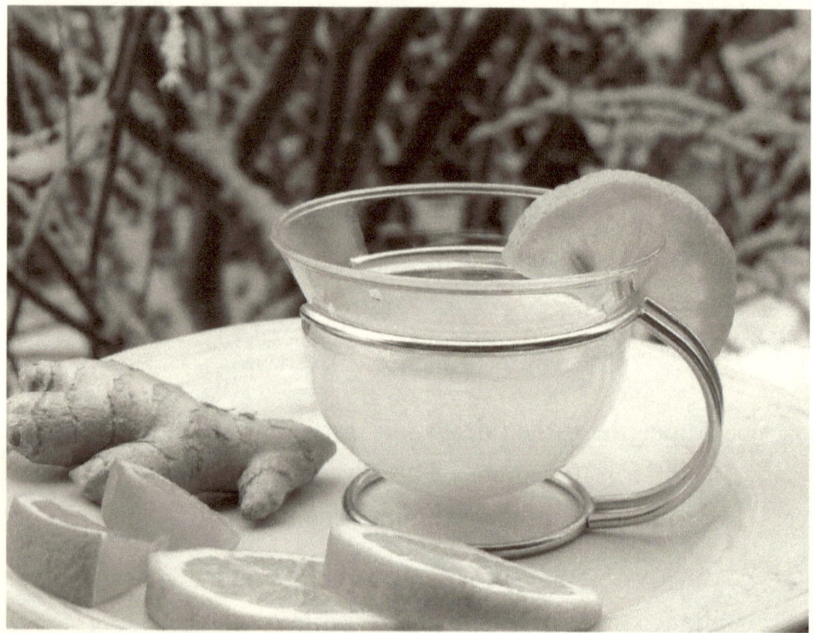

A switchel is a refreshing and invigorating drink that is made from apple cider vinegar and is also known as a switchel. It contains tons of probiotics that will help with digestion and gut health, plus it contains ample vitamin C and other immune-boosting vitamins from the lemon in it! This drink is the perfect addition to your morning routine to rev up your daily immunity, or it can be enjoyed anytime as a refreshing pick-me-up!

Ingredients

4 slices ginger

3 ¾ cups water, divided

2 tablespoons apple cider vinegar (like Braggs – "with the mother in it") more to taste

Juice of ½ –1 lemon (or sublimes or other citrus! Blood oranges work well too!)

1 tablespoon honey (preferably raw) or maple syrup or stevia to taste -optional, depending on how sweet you like it.

Directions

1. Place ginger in one cup of water in a small pot and bring to a boil. Let cool (proper cooling is very important to ensure that the heat doesn't kill the healthy bacteria in the apple cider vinegar or honey that is added in step 2)

2. Pour the ginger water, remaining water, apple cider vinegar, the juice from half a lemon, and your choice of sweetener into a quart mason jar. Stir and adjust lemon and sweetness to your taste.

3. Store in a pitcher or mason jar, either in the fridge or at room temp (if you intend to drink water throughout the day).

4. Enjoy first thing in the morning to aid the liver in cleansing, enhancing your immunity, or in the afternoon for an energizing pick-me-up.

5. This drink will keep in the fridge for one week.

WARM WINTER SALAD

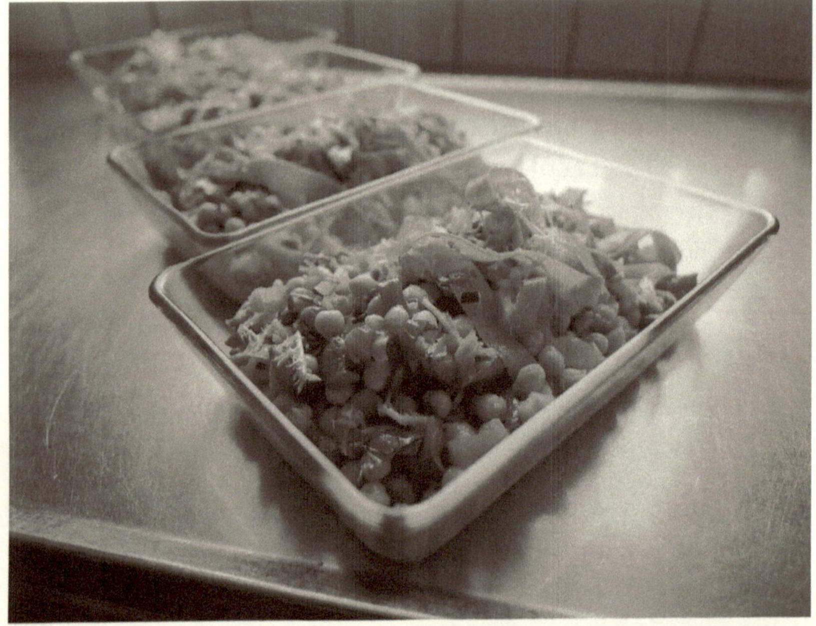

This warm salad is baked in the oven on a sheet pan, making it both easy and delicious! It contains a wide variety of different vegetables that are filled with tons of vitamins and minerals plus lots of fiber to help with healthy digestion. This salad can be eaten as an entree or as a side dish and saves well in the fridge to be eaten as leftovers throughout the week.

Ingredients

1 head cauliflower, cut into small florets

2-3 large carrots (or parsnips), peeled and cut into 1 inch thick pieces

1 fennel bulb, cored and cut in 1/3 inch thick wedges

1 red onion, sliced into 1/2 inch wedges

14-ounce of canned chickpeas (rinsed, drained, and patted dry)

2-3 tablespoons olive oil

2 garlic cloves, finely minced

2 teaspoons coriander

2 teaspoons sumac (optional, but tasty)

1 teaspoon salt

1/2 teaspoon cracked pepper

zest from one lemon

Couple handfuls of baby spinach

Tahini Sauce (thinned out with a little water, to make it more like a dressing)

3-4 tablespoons Dukkah (or a 2 tablespoons Zaatar)

3-4 tablespoons fresh dill

A teaspoon of lemon juice

Chili flakes

Directions

1. Preheat oven to 425F.

2. Place the cauliflower florets, carrots, fennel, onion, and chickpeas in an EXTRA large bowl. Toss with the olive oil, minced garlic, coriander, salt, pepper, and lemon zest. Toss well.

3. Place in a single layer on one or two parchment-lined sheet pans. Bake for 15 minutes, then toss veggies and rotate pans. Bake 10-15 minutes more until the cauliflower is tender and edges crispy.

4. If serving on the sheet pan, move all the veggies onto one pan. Spread around evenly. Top with the baby spinach, drizzle the tahini sauce over the top (diagonally is nice), and sprinkle with the Dukkah. Squeeze with a little lemon.

5. Garnish with fresh dill and Chili flakes.

Enjoy!

TURMERIC GINGER MUFFINS

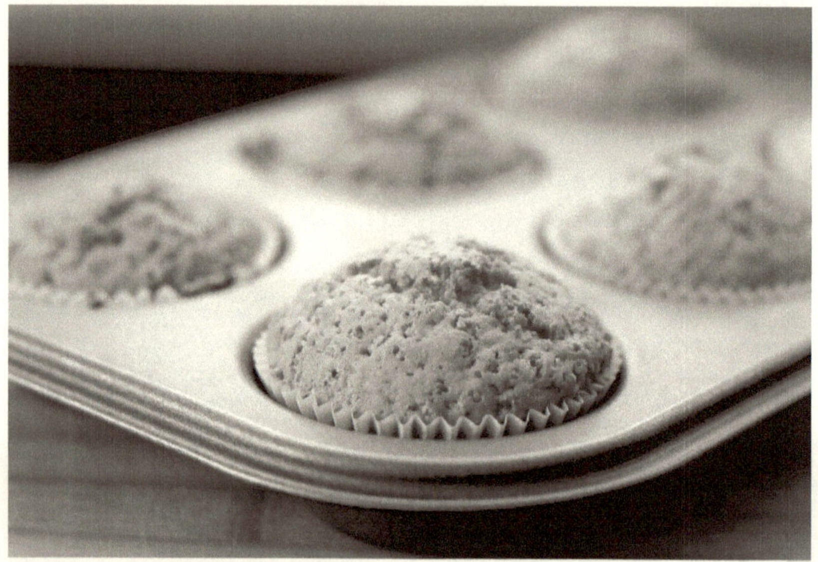

These muffins combine turmeric's anti-inflammatory effects with ginger's antiviral effects to create a delicious snack packed full of nutrients. These muffins make a great breakfast, mid-day snack, or dessert that will help keep your immune system strong any time of the year but especially during cold and flu season.

Ingredients

1 3/4 cup oat flour*

1 1/2 tsp baking powder

1/2 tsp baking soda

1/2 tsp salt

1 1/2 tsp cinnamon

1 tsp ginger

1 tsp turmeric

1 cup ripe mashed banana

1/2 cup coconut sugar

1/4 cup coconut oil melted and slightly cooled

1/2 cup almond milk

1 tsp vanilla

2 organic eggs

3/4 cup rolled oats

Garnish with additional coconut sugar and rolled oats

Optional

Directions

1. Preheat oven to 350 degrees, and spray muffin tin with nonstick coconut oil or avocado spray.

2. In a medium mixing bowl, add all dry ingredients and whisk together - oat flour, baking powder, baking soda, salt, cinnamon, turmeric, and ginger.

3. In a separate large bowl, add all wet ingredients - melted coconut oil, mashed banana, coconut sugar, almond milk, vanilla, and eggs, whisk until well combined.

4. Add dry ingredients to wet ingredients and stir them together until just mixed.

5. Fold in rolled oats.

6. Divide into 12 grease muffins, approximately 1/4 cup batter in each.

7. Garnish with extra rolled oats and coconut sugar if desired, then bake 17-18 minutes or until the toothpick inserted comes out clean.

Enjoy!

IMMUNE BOOSTING GINGER TEA

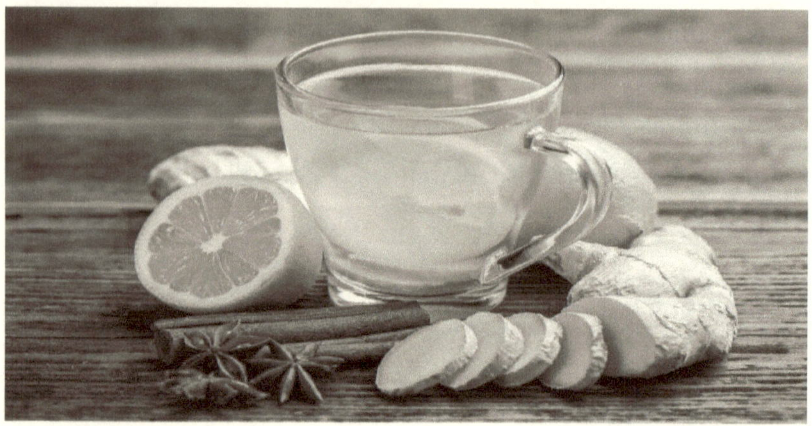

This is a great tea that you should make to protect yourself against not only COVID 19 and other coronavirus, but also the flu. This is because the ingredients in this tea will boost your immune defense against these viruses and will also help to arrest the symptoms of these viruses should you contract them. The Vitamin C in the lemon will help to kill any corona or flu virus that has invaded your body. The ginger will reduce the inflammation of your lungs and help you to breath more easily. Adding honey will sooth your throat and reduce coughing and the cayenne pepper will help to keep your blood vessels open so that you get adequate oxygen flowing throughout your respiratory system. Cinnamon is not only a good alternative to sugar. It is also known to prevent blood clots. It can also be used an anti-inflammatory. It improves heart health and improves blood circulation. So added it to this tea does a lot more than you think.

Ingredients

1 cup water

1-inch ginger root

1/2 a lemon

Cinnamon bark

Honey (optional)

Cayenne pepper (optional)

Directions

1. Peel (optional) and grate a 1-inch piece of fresh ginger root

2. Add the juice of half a lemon

3. Add a stick of cinnamon

4. Boil one cup of water and pour into the ginger and lemon

5. Leave to infuse for 5-10 minutes

6. Strain into your favorite cup/mug

7. Serve with some honey or cayenne pepper (completely optional).

MATCHA AND PINEAPPLE SMOOTHIE

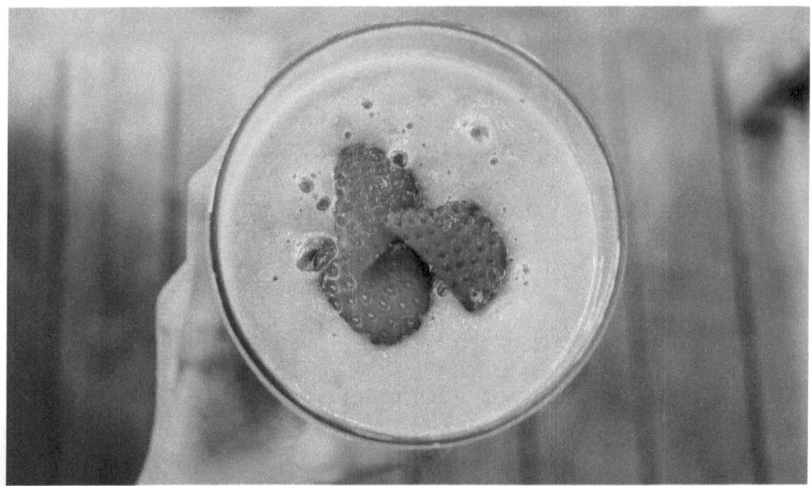

Matcha is a type of finely ground green tea, and it is filled with so many vitamins, minerals, and antioxidants. When combined with the sweet and tropical pineapple fruit, this smoothing is brimming with lots of immune-boosting properties and digestive enzymes to improve your gut health. On top of all this, it is refreshing and delicious!

Ingredients

1 banana

1 C fresh pineapple

1 C kale or spinach

½ teaspoon matcha powder, plus more to taste

½ cup nut or soy milk

squeeze of lemon

A handful of ice cubes (or you can use frozen bananas instead!)

Directions

Blend all in a blender until very smooth.

Enjoy!!

THE ORANGE SMOOTHIE

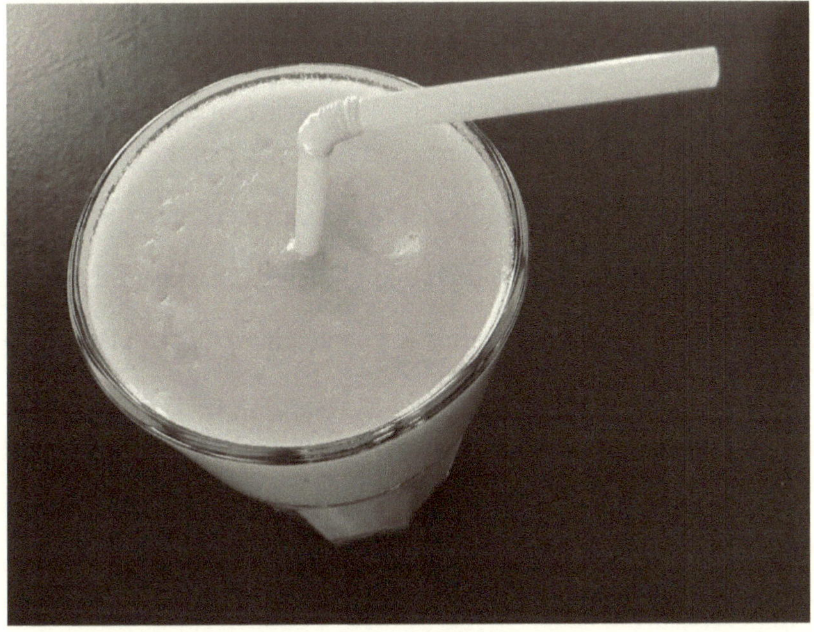

If this smoothie's bright orange color isn't enough to make your mouth water, then the superfoods that it contains within it should do the trick! This smoothie is perfect for breakfast or a snack, especially during cold and flu season when your immune system could use some added help!

Ingredients

1 Carrot

1 Orange

8 oz apple juice or coconut milk

1 apple

1 kiwi

1 tbs apple cider vinegar

1 very small finger of ginger optional

1. Add apple juice or coconut milk to your blender. (Apple juice will make the smoothie sweeter.)

2. Peel your orange and cut in half place in the blender. Cut the apple in half and remove seeds place in the blender.

3. Remove skin from Kiwi and place in blender.

4. Add apple cider vinegar and a small piece of peeled ginger.

5. Chop your carrot into a few large chunks, then place them in the blender.

6. Blend for about 3 minutes or until smooth. You can add more apple juice or coconut milk for desired thickness.

Enjoy!

BLUEBERRY BANANA SMOOTHIE BOWL

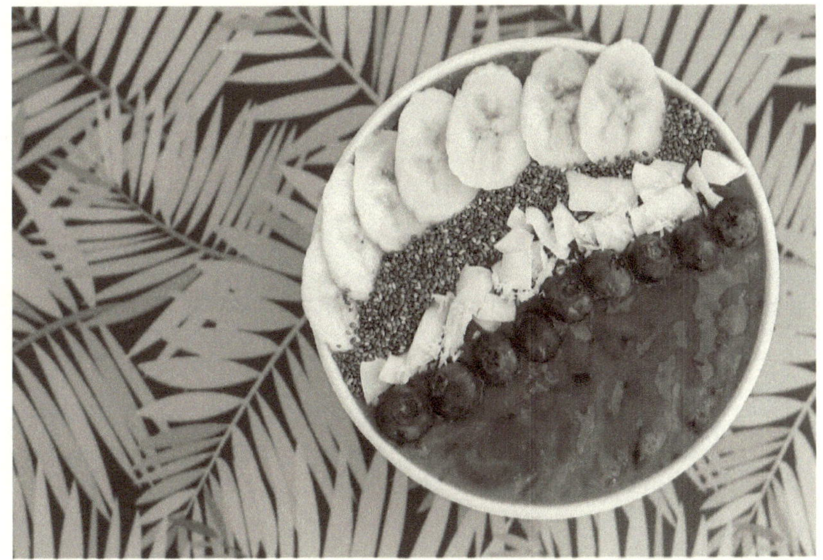

What better way to start your day than with a delicious and nutritious smoothie bowl. This blueberry banana smoothie bowl contains tons of vitamin C to help fight off infection, plus loads of antioxidants and immune-boosting superfoods to help keep you healthy and full of energy.

Ingredients

½ cup almond milk

1 cup frozen blueberry

2 tbsp raw cacao powder

2 tbsp honey

¼ medium avocado

1 large frozen banana

½ cup ice

fresh blueberries

pumpkin seeds

hemp seeds

goji berries

chopped Brazil nuts

Directions

1. Place the milk, honey, avocado, and cocoa powder in a high-power blender and process until smooth.

2. Add the frozen blueberries, banana, and ice and process until thick and creamy.

3. Transfer the smoothie to a bowl and top with fresh blueberries, pumpkin seeds, goji berries, hemp seeds, and chopped Brazil nuts or your favorite toppings.

Enjoy!

IMMUNE GUMMIES

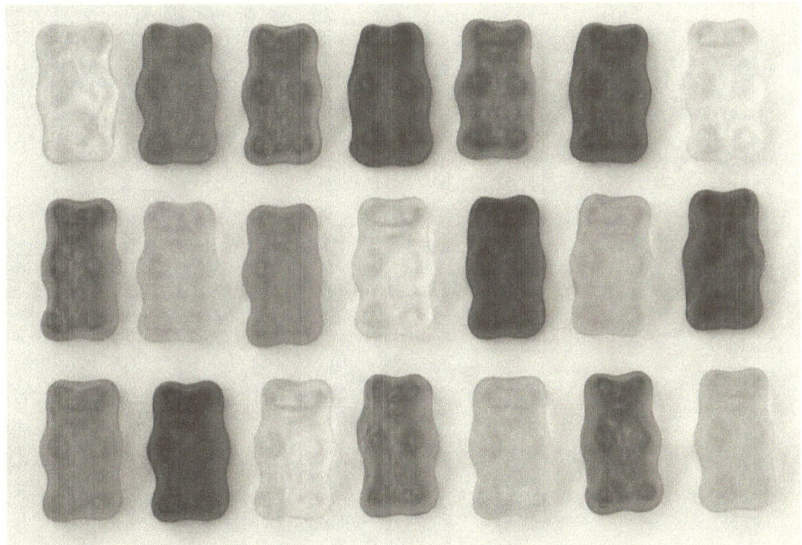

If you are looking for a quick and easy way to get some virus-fighting goodness, then why not try making these delicious and easy immune-supporting gummies. They are packed full of vitamin C, antioxidants, antiviral and antibacterial ingredients that will help you keep healthy all throughout the cold and flu season.

Ingredients

¾ cup lemon juice

3 tbsp raw honey

½ cup grass-fed gelatin

1 cup hot water

½ cup room temperature water

1 tbsp cinnamon

3 inches of ginger

1. In a small saucepan, boil 1 cup of water on high heat.

2. Once boiled, remove from heat and allow the water to cool down completely.

3. Add in the gelatin and whisk well.

4. Next, add the lemon, ginger, cinnamon, and ½ cup of water to a high-speed blender. Blend on high until the mixture is smooth.

5. Slowly add the mixture to the water and gelatin.

6. Once the mixture has cooled, add in the raw honey and mix until well combined.

7. Pour the mixture into molds and place it in the fridge for approximately two hours.

8. Pop-out of molds and store in a cool place.

Enjoy!

Afterword

As you can see, our immunity is a complex system that relies on the proper balance of multiple different factors in order for it to protect us from attack and to keep us free from disease.

A healthy diet filled with a variety of whole foods combined with a regular exercise plan will help keep our gut healthy, provide us with the nutrients that our bodies need to function properly and efficiently and help keep our weight in check. Suppose we combine this with a lifestyle that minimizes toxins (including alcohol and tobacco), provides us with plenty of sleep, keeps us hydrated, and allows us to manage our level of stress effectively. If we are able to do this, we will be able to give our immune systems the further support that it requires.

Finally, if we boost our immunity with added supplements and therapies, we will be better able to live longer, healthier lives.

Our bodies are miraculous machines that work hard for us every day, keeping us safe from pathogens and giving us vibrant health and longevity. With a little effort and care, we can provide them with the added assistance they need to continue working hard for us and protecting us from future illness.

Final Thought

I would like to thank you for purchasing and taking the time to read this book. I am highly honored that you did and I sincerely hope that your life will indeed be better off for doing so. If you did indeed find this book to be informative and potentially life changing, I would greatly appreciate your taking five minutes of your precious time to go on Amazon or the Kindle book store and leave a review. Let others know what you thought of this book.

In my next book I am going to show you how you can optimize your overall health which in turn will increase your longevity.

Lastly, I would like to invite you to join my Facebook group[1] where you can interact with other readers of this book. I and others also post a lot of information about natural health, the immune system, emotional wellbeing, herbal remedies, healing foods, diets and exercise routines. I created the group to provide my readers and additional resource that they can use to find answers to any questions that they may have about their health. So, I hope to see you there.

Once again thank you SO MUCH for choosing to read this book and I hope that you will give me the privilege of serving you in the future.

www.amazon.com/ryp